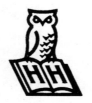

HERE'S LOOKING AT YOU, KID!

An Owl Book
HENRY HOLT AND COMPANY
New York

HERE'S LOOKING AT YOU, KID!

A
Busy Parent's Guide
to Children's Grooming,
Health, and Clothing Basics

CAROL STRALEY

Henry Holt and Company, Inc.
Publishers since 1866
115 West 18th Street
New York, New York 10011

Henry Holt® is a registered
trademark of Henry Holt and Company, Inc.

Copyright © 1993 by Carol Straley
All rights reserved.
Published in Canada by Fitzhenry & Whiteside Ltd.,
91 Granton Drive, Richmond Hill, Ontario L4B 2N5.

Library of Congress Cataloging-in-Publication Data
Straley, Carol.
Here's looking at you, kid! / Carol Straley.—1st Owl Book ed.
p. cm.
Includes bibliographical references.
1. Grooming for boys. 2. Grooming for girls. 3. Children—Health
and hygiene. 4. Beauty, Personal. 5. Child rearing. I. Title.
RA777.S83   1993   92-45815
646.7'046—dc20   CIP

ISBN 0-8050-2048-9 (An Owl Book: pbk.)

First Edition—1993

Designed by Katy Riegel
Illustrations by Linda Johnson Azzara

Printed in the United States of America
All first editions are printed on acid-free paper. ∞

1   3   5   7   9   10   8   6   4   2

To my parents, Philomena and George, who taught me that beauty is truth and showed me the importance of love and good humor in caring for children.

To James, whose love and devotion keep me going and whose own creative spirit inspires me to pursue my craft.

Contents

	Author's Note	xi
	Foreword	xiii
	Acknowledgments	xv
	Introduction	1
1	Skin Deep: Help for Healthy Skin	5
2	Rub-a-Dub-Dub: Tips for the Tub	34
3	Bites, Bumps, and Sunburn: Skin Care for the Great Outdoors	53
4	Hair Today: Tips for Shining Hair and a Healthy Scalp	72
5	Hair Shape-up: How to Cut, Curl, and Style Your Child's Hair	89
6	Smile! Dental Care for Your Child's Teeth and Gums	111
7	Eyes Right! Eye Care and Eye Wear for Kids	139
8	Clothes-Smart: Year-Round Guide to No-Fuss Dressing	171
	Bibliography	197
	Index	199

Author's Note

While much of the information in this book is medically based, it is not intended to take the place of consulting your doctor. All of the information in this book has been checked for accuracy with the proper authorities. However, differences of opinion among physicians are inevitable, and your own doctor or health care expert may suggest an alternative course of treatment. Please consult your pediatrician for all matters concerning your child's health.

Although I have mentioned many items by brand name in this book, I am not endorsing any particular products. While I have personally found the products mentioned to be excellent, sensitivity to any substance is individual. Again, please seek the advice of your pediatrician when selecting products for your child.

Foreword

Carol Straley has produced an invaluable guide that all parents can use to help their children achieve two important and related goals: feeling good on the inside and looking good to the world outside. Drawing on her long experience as a beauty and health editor, as well as on relevant published literature and the wisdom of both parents and professionals, she provides insightful advice not only in the management of everyday tasks such as bathing and dressing, but in the resolution of crises ranging from skin rashes in newborns to crooked teeth in preadolescence. The book will be a rich source of information and comfort for mothers and fathers of infants, toddlers, and school-age children.

The importance of this book, however, extends beyond the detailed guidance it offers. For in adopting the author's specific tactics for helping children in matters of hygiene and appearance, parents will be embracing a vital strategy for building self-esteem in their young. How children learn to view themselves—how worthy and likable they feel they are—can be colored significantly by their sense of physical well-being and the images they have of their own bodies. Moreover, the link between body image and self-esteem is often reinforced by social experience. Studies in social psychology have shown that children perceived as physically pleasing tend to be highly regarded by both their peers and teachers. For better or worse, the world is indeed "looking at you, kid."

The author offers her sane and empathic guidance without in any way fostering an obsessional concern about matters of physical care and grooming. Instead this book appeals to our most wholesome impulses to care for our children—keep them healthy, heal their hurts, enhance their appearance, and, ultimately, help them navigate on their own the tasks of self-care and grooming that are such a vital part of our lives.

—JULIUS SEGAL, PH.D., author
of *A Child's Journey: Faces that Shape the Lives of Our Young*,
and former director, office of Scientific Information,
National Institute of Mental Health

Acknowledgments

The realization of this book has truly been a team effort. I would especially like to thank: Madeleine Morel, my smart and savvy agent, for believing in me; Theresa Burns, my editor, for her unflagging enthusiasm and creative direction; and Pam Abrams, my coworker, for sending the opportunity to write this book to my door.

Heartfelt thanks also go to my colleagues at *Parents* magazine, in particular: Ann Pleshette Murphy, editor-in-chief, for her generous support; Carole Horii, creative director, for having very strong shoulders to lean on; and Virginia Fisher, my assistant, for always being on the lookout for useful information.

I am also grateful to my dear friends: Kathleen Raines, for sharing her wise and witty parenting strategies; Valerie Monroe, for always listening and providing much-appreciated reality checks; and Lisa Fournier, for understanding what it takes to meet deadlines. A fond thank you also goes to Jessie Turberg, for the nurturing power of her wisdom and caring.

This book would also not have been possible without the help of many health care professionals who gave freely of their time, energy, and expertise. Along with the doctors and scientists mentioned in the

Acknowledgments

text, I would like to thank the following: Patricia Agin, Ph.D., project team manager of research and development, pharmaceuticals and toiletries in the Schering-Plough Healthcare Products Division; John Bogert, D.D.S., executive director, American Academy of Pediatric Dentistry; Ron Di Salvo, Ph.D., director of research and product development for John Paul Mitchell Systems; T.M. Graber, D.M.D., M.S.D., and Ph.D., editor, *American Journal of Pediatric Dentistry;* David Hansen, O.D., pediatric optometry consultant, American Optometric Association; Bradford R. Katchen, M.D., assistant attending and clinical instructor of dermatology at Beth Israel Medical Center, New York City; Suzanne M. Levine, D.P.M., adjunct faculty member of the New York College of Medicine, Wycoff Hospital, Forest Hills, New York; Zenona W. Mally, M.D., clinical assistant professor of dermatology at Georgetown University Department of Medicine, Washington, D.C.; Stephen C. Miller, O.D., director, Clinical Care Center, American Optometric Association; Michael Pier, O.D., director of clinical research at Bausch & Lomb; Larry R. Price, D.D.S., who practices in El Paso, Texas; and Charles Zugerman, M.D., associate professor of clinical dermatology at Northwestern University Medical School, Chicago.

I would also like to thank the communications coordinators and editors of the various professional organizations who provided me with the latest health care information, put me in touch with many of the doctors I interviewed for this book, and reviewed parts of the manuscript: Lucy Kavaler of the Skin Cancer Foundation; Ann Marie Lopes of the National Safe Kids Campaign; Irene Malbin of the Cosmetics, Toiletries, and Fragrances Association; Maureen Geyton of the American Academy of Pediatrics; Amy Fox of the American Academy of Pediatric Dentistry; the Contact Lens Council; and Charlotte A. Rancilio of the American Optometric Association.

I also appreciate the efforts of the following publicists, communications managers, and executives who kept me up-to-date with information on children's health and grooming products, clothes, and accessories: Frances R. Stelz for Marchon & Marcolin Eyewear; Richard Kase, manager, public relations, Bausch & Lomb; Kelly Ann Sherry for Bausch & Lomb; Mauri Edwards for the Sunglass Association of America; Leslie R. Resnik for Sears Optical; Dave Furman and Laurie Brackett for Stride-Rite; Alice Fixx for Tsumura,

Acknowledgments

Inc.; Susan Handy for Mennen; Giora Davidovits and Larry Kagel for Biological Rescue Products, Inc.; Susan Jones for Kids at Large; Kim Grady and Lisa Moll Byelick for The Athlete's Foot; Christel Henke for OshKosh B'Gosh; Marcie Grossman for Sears; and Lisa Anderson for Cotton, Incorporated.

Special thanks go to Arlene Benza, public relations director for Nubest Salon, for all her help in coordinating the information on children's haircuts.

For sharing their knowledge on children's clothing I would like to thank the following fashion experts: Chris Blake of OshKosh B'Gosh; Cassandra Muller of Wippette Kids; Kim Runyon, cofounder of Kids at Large; Ernie Lippman of Sears; Roy Jamrog and Laurie Sentor of Stride-Rite; and Tom Brunick, director of The Athlete's Foot Wear Test Center.

Introduction

YOUR CHILD'S LOOKS matter. While not in the same realm as kindness, talent, imagination, and intellectual gifts, your child's appearance is way up there on the list of things that count as sources of self-esteem.

As your children grow up, you want them to be proud of their achievements and abilities. You also want them to feel good about the way they look. This does not mean that your child has to look as if she stepped out of the glossy pages of a fashion magazine. And it has less to do with having a pert nose and straight teeth than with feeling confident and at ease with oneself.

As a parent you play a major role in helping your child develop a healthy perspective on his or her looks. You also help your child learn the basics of grooming, hygiene, and dressing—big steps on the journey toward independence and self-reliance.

Whether you are changing a diaper for the first time or taking your child to get braces, you're in charge of your child's good looks and good health. And this can be a challenge even for the most patient parent. You may be fast becoming an expert in sibling rivalry and the terrible twos. But what do you do if your baby gets a sunburn? How can you help your young nail-nibbler break the habit? What do you do when your child comes home from nursery school with head lice?

That's where *Here's Looking at You, Kid!* comes in. This book was created to answer the many questions on health care and grooming that can boggle a busy parent's mind.

When I became beauty editor of *Parents* magazine eight years ago, moms and dads began to ask for my advice on a myriad of topics concerning their children's hygiene and head-to-toe grooming. "How can I get the tangles out of my daughter's hair?" "How can I persuade my toddler to take his bath?" "Is it safe to use a children's sunscreen on an infant?"

This barrage of questions was posed by sophisticated adults who were well versed in many of the aspects of child care. Like you, they'd pored over all the baby books in the pursuit of polishing their parenting skills. And yet there were a few gaps where Dr. Spock and other child-rearing experts left off—such as help on how to get a fussy toddler to brush his teeth; how to choose safe, gentle grooming products; what it takes to make a child feel more confident about getting glasses or wearing braces.

The questions also gave me a more accurate reading of what it takes to be a parent. You have to be ready to treat the minor medical mishaps that may not need a doctor's care but still require prompt attention. You need the know-how to teach your child good grooming. And you need smart strategies to outwit all the maneuvers your child can create to avoid taking a bath or getting dressed in the morning!

As I considered this, I began to see the need for a children's health and grooming guide. After talking to many parents hungry for information on everything from tear-free shampooing to hassle-free shoe shopping, I felt that it would be helpful to have one book that solves many of the health care, grooming, and dressing problems that can challenge today's parents. The result is *Here's Looking at You, Kid!*

In order to put together a one-stop resource of helpful hints and up-to-the-minute information, I consulted many of the top specialists in the health, grooming, and clothing professions. Their suggestions and guidelines will help to make light work of many of your daily child care tasks.

Introduction

Writing this book was also a wonderful opportunity to draw from my eighteen years of experience as a beauty and health editor. My own expertise, my conversations with resourceful, imaginative parents, and countless interviews with the experts—all helped me to arrive at the tips and tricks that will enable your child to look and feel his best.

On these pages you'll find information on basic health care, home remedies for insect bites, bee stings, and more, as well as recipes to whip up tub treats for your child's bath. You'll find on-the-spot advice for coping with such minidisasters as getting chewing gum out of your child's hair or nail polish out of her clothes, and quick fixes for spills or stains, from fingerpaint to grape juice.

This book will also help you lower the cost of children's haircuts with step-by-step plans for trimming your child's hair. And you'll learn how to teach your child to wash his hair, floss his teeth, keep nails neat, and more.

For those times that put your parenting to the test, there is help on taking the anxiety out of your child's visits to the dentist, tips on stress-less dressing—such as how to outfox a fidgety toddler—and guidelines on boosting your child's confidence and helping her to evolve a healthy self-image.

Here's Looking at You, Kid! is directed to parents of children from birth to twelve years of age because of the shifts in grooming and health care needs that come about as children grow up. Babies and toddlers are, naturally, dependent on your full-time tender, loving care. At two years of age, a child can begin to take the first steps in self-care, such as learning to brush his teeth and wash his face. And by the time a child is three or four years old, she may be more eager to have a hand in her grooming. She may want to rub soap on her tummy during her bath or run her fingers through the shampoo suds. But at this stage, a young child can't reach his back teeth with a toothbrush, scrub his back, or rinse out shampoo lather. You're still on call to take over when needed.

By the time your child is about six or seven years of age, she will become more independent. She has mastered the skills of getting dressed and tying her shoelaces. She can also handle many aspects of her grooming on her own, such as showering and shampooing and scrubbing her nails. In fact, she may not want you to have any say at all! But children at this age don't always make grooming a priority, and you will still have to step in to remind them to brush their teeth (and to make sure they've done a thorough job!) or dress warmly on a bone-chilling day. And while preteens are busy at self-expression and honing emerging identities, they still need your help. This is the age when many youngsters begin to wear braces or trade in glasses for contact lenses.

Here's Looking at You, Kid! will help to coach you through all the stages of your child's changing health care and grooming needs. I hope you find that it is a book you can count on to solve many of the sticky situations that are bound to come up as your child grows up. Whether you have a newborn, toddler, or school-age child, you're sure to find many of the answers you need to make many of your everyday child care decisions. And as you improve your expertise, your child will learn the good health and grooming habits that will last a lifetime.

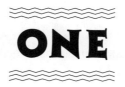

ONE

Skin Deep: Help for Healthy Skin

WHAT IS MORE delightful to the touch than the soft, tender skin of a child? The smooth, fragrant skin you love to nuzzle up to is also one of the largest organs of the body and serves as your child's remarkable defense against injury and infection. Like a large, protective envelope, the skin holds in body fluids, shields the internal organs against damage, and defends against invading bacteria.

The skin also works like a thermostat to regulate body temperature. (Sweat glands in the skin produce perspiration, which cools the body as it evaporates; layers of fat in the deepest layer of the skin conserve heat.) And touch receptors in the skin respond to pressure (such as your loving caress), temperature, and other changes in our environment, then quickly send these messages to the brain. The skin metabolizes vitamin D, renews itself constantly, and when injured, sends its efficient repair system into action to mend the damage.

This chapter will take you through the basics of caring for your child's skin. It will show you how to baby your newborn's skin and how to safely treat common skin care problems, from diaper rash to eczema. You'll learn how to choose gentle soaps, lotions, and powders and how to spot potential irritants in skin care products.

There are soothers for cold sores and chapped lips, remedies for chapped hands, and basic first aid for cuts and scrapes. Tips on nail care, including cures for nail biting, will keep your child looking neat and well groomed down to his fingertips and toes!

THE BASICS OF HEALTHY SKIN

While you may be most concerned with the way your child's skin looks, it is a good idea to understand how this highly complex system works. The skin is composed of three layers: the *epidermis*, which is the thin outer layer; the *dermis*, the middle layer; and the *subcutaneous* tissue level, which is the deepest layer of the skin.

The epidermis generates plump, healthy new skin cells and produces *melanin*, the pigment that colors the skin. As they mature, the new cells push upward. By the time these cells reach the surface they die, becoming flat and dry. The skin that feels so irresistibly soft is actually a lifeless protein called *keratin*. Eventually these dead cells are sloughed off and replaced with a new supply.

The dermis, which nourishes and supports the epidermis, is made up of a network of *collagen* and *elastin*, fibrous proteins that give the skin its strength and elasticity. (One reason why a child's skin is so much smoother and firmer than adult skin is that the fibers of collagen and elastin are fresh; time has not weakened them, and they have also not been subjected to years of sun damage, which causes collagen and elastin to collapse.) The dermis contains the oil glands, hair follicles, muscle tissue, sweat glands, nerve fibers, and blood vessels. And it supplies skin cells with water to keep skin smooth and supple. (Your child's skin doesn't feel as taut and dry as a mature adult's because the natural water content is higher.) The deepest level of the skin contains more blood vessels and nerve fibers. This is where fat cells are stored, to insulate the body against cold and to act as a shock absorber.

While it is durable and washable, young skin is also delicate, sensitive, and vulnerable to irritation. At any age, your child's skin needs protection from overexposure to the elements and irritants in both the indoor and outdoor environment. After all, your child is born with smooth, soft skin—and you want to keep it that way.

TLC FOR NEWBORN SKIN

If you are the parent of a newborn, you know that your baby's skin needs extra tender loving care. Because it has not developed completely, the skin of a newborn is not yet fully efficient as a protective barrier against external harm. For example, melanin, which gives the skin a small amount of natural protection against sun damage, is not fully developed at birth. It also takes time for your baby's sweat glands, oil glands, and hair follicles to develop completely. Minor imperfections are normal.

Tiny white or yellow papules called *milia*, which look like whiteheads, may show up on an infant's cheeks, nose, and chin. They are symptoms of undeveloped or blocked sweat glands. Milia need no special treatment and will disappear within three or four weeks.

Within a few days after birth, many infants develop a splotchy rash on the back, chest, or face. This condition, *toxic erythema*, is often referred to as newborn rash. But don't let the word *toxic* worry you. While the exact cause is unknown (some doctors think it may be a temporary reaction to heat), newborn rash is harmless, requires no treatment, and usually clears up within ten days.

Thin and delicate, a newborn's skin is also easily penetrated by the ingredients in products that touch the skin. To play it safe, the American Academy of Dermatology advises that you check with your pediatrician before applying any skin care product or medication to your newborn's skin.

Keep in mind that an infant's sensitive skin is also easily sunburned. To protect your baby's skin, take the advice of the American Academy of Dermatolology and The Skin Cancer Foundation and keep your infant out of direct sunlight. (For more on sun protection, see chapter 3.) Even a moderate dose of midday sunshine can result in a nasty sunburn, which can harm your baby's health. (Dehydration, fever, faintness, delirium, shock, dangerously low blood pressure, and irregular heartbeat are among the dangers of too much sun.) Treat sunburn in a baby under the age of one year as an emergency and call your doctor immediately.

Always make sure that a baby's bathwater is not too hot. To be safe, the temperature should range from 90 to 95 degrees F for a comfortably tepid bath and 96 to 100 degrees F for a mildly warm bath. For an accurate measurement, use a liquid crystal bath thermometer. Or swish your hand up to your wrist in the water. (For more safety tips on bathing, see chapter 2.)

Never drink hot liquids while holding your baby. One wrong move and your drink can spill, scalding both you and your baby. Steer clear of any hot liquids, heated appliances, or other hot objects whenever caring for your baby.

Don't smoke while handling your baby. There's always the risk of burning her with your cigarette. (You should consider quitting smoking. Any cigarette smoke your baby inhales can irritate her lungs and jeopardize her health. This goes for children at any age.)

BABY'S SKIN CARE SUPPLIES

When it comes to choosing products to keep baby's skin clean, smooth, and healthy, less is more. A few basics will go a long way to pamper and protect your little one's birthday suit. Coming up, a checklist of what to keep on hand for baby's everyday skin care needs:

- Mild, unscented baby soap or gentle soap-free cleanser
- Rubbing alcohol
- Sterile cotton balls
- Flexible cotton swabs
- Pediatrician-recommended diaper rash ointment
- Baby powder
- Baby lotion and/or baby oil
- Baby wipes

While most of the items on this list are basic, you may need some help in selecting others. The following guidelines will help you to choose the best products for your baby.

Baby Soaps and Cleansers

For protection against moisture loss, choose special baby soaps and cleansers formulated with skin-softening emollients. Because fragrances and colorants are potentially irritating, baby soaps should also be unscented and dye-free.

Transparent baby soaps are made with glycerine, a clear, fatty liquid that attracts moisture. One wonderful advantage of glycerine soaps: they are formulated to rinse off easily. Any soap film that remains on the skin is drying and may irritate sensitive skin. So whatever soap or cleanser you choose, be sure to rinse your baby thoroughly—and to use your soap or cleanser sparingly.

Baby Powder

A light application of baby powder helps to absorb excess moisture. It also helps to minimize the chafing that comes from baby's clothes and diapers rubbing against bare skin.

Some doctors recommend a talc-free formula. Current medical evidence shows that inhaling airborne powder can cause a baby to have breathing problems. The fine particles of talc can irritate the lungs and cause an inflammatory reaction, which may trigger wheezing, coughing, labored breathing, and vomiting. If your baby accidentally inhales talcum powder, sit him up and give him some water or milk. If this doesn't help, bring your baby to the nearest hospital emergency room.

Some experts believe that cornstarch does a better job of soaking up wetness than powders with talc. This is because talcum powder repels water, while cornstarch absorbs moisture. You can now get baby powders that contain finely milled oatmeal at your drugstore or supermarket. Baby powders with skin-soothing maize and rice bran are available in specialty shops, such as The Body Shop, which feature products made with plant extracts and herbs. All of these formulas are said to be extra absorbent. They also cause less dusting in the air.

Whatever formula you choose, the key to applying baby powder safely is to use it sparingly. Do not shake the powder freely onto baby's skin or near her face. Your baby might breathe in the loose puffs of powder that float in the air. The safest method: simply sprinkle a little in your hand and gently smooth it over desired areas. Also, be sure to keep baby powder tightly capped and out of baby's reach when not in use.

Baby Lotions and Baby Oils

To soften any dry, flaky patches on baby's skin, you may want to smooth on a little baby lotion or baby oil. Many baby lotions and oils available today have been dermatologist-tested and shown to be mild and safe. However, pediatric dermatologists point out that mineral oil (particularly undiluted mineral oil) has been known to result in *folliculitis*, an inflammation of the hair follicles. Sometimes, if a greasy film is left on baby's skin, the oil blocks the pores (openings on the surface of the skin) leading to the hair follicles, and a pimply red rash may flare up. Your child can also get a heat rash if the oil occludes the sweat ducts.

If you prefer not to use rich or heavy oils, there are so-called "light" versions, such as Baby Magic Lite Baby Oil, formulated to be absorbed more quickly. A more refined, lighter grade of mineral oil is used along with an ingredient called *cyclo-methicone*, which helps to speed up the absorption of oil into the skin. Since they are less greasy, light oils may lessen the chances of getting folliculitis.

You can also find baby lotions and oils made without mineral oil. These formulas may contain vegetable oils, such as soya oil, which are more refined than mineral oil. (Mustela Extra Mild Moisturizing Lotion, available at Caswell-Massey shops, is made with sweet almond oil.) Or they may contain plant-based ingredients such as aloe vera and chamomile extracts, soothing ingredients that help to calm irritated skin. You can find these formulas in shops that offer naturally based skin care products. No matter what lotion or oil you choose, apply it sparingly and discontinue use at the first sign of irritation.

Petroleum Jelly

Chances are that your parents kept a jar of petroleum jelly in the family medicine cabinet when you were growing up and that you've been using the stuff to take off your eye makeup and soften chapped lips long before the arrival of your first baby. Petroleum jelly is a favorite standby of many parents—and doctors—because it forms a thick protective film on the skin. Because it is water-resistant, petroleum jelly is often used to prevent diaper rash. It also works well to relieve minor skin irritations.

If you like the barrier action of petroleum jelly but prefer something that is not as thick for your baby (or older child), try a petrolatum-free vegetable jelly. Vegetable oils such as sunflower oil, safflower oil, and olive oil take the place of petrolatum, making the jelly lighter and less greasy. Vegetable jelly is also free of pore-clogging mineral oil.

Baby Wipes

Formulated to quickly and neatly cleanse the diaper area, commercial baby wipes are disposable tissues infused with a mild skin cleanser. They can also be used for quick cleanups of the hands and face. As handy as baby wipes are, they can add up to a big expense if used with every diaper change. But because they are portable, you may want to stash a pack in your diaper bag when you take baby on the road. Baby wipes with moisturizing ingredients such as aloe vera or chamomile extract are especially soothing. As with any baby skin care product, discontinue use if baby's skin becomes irritated.

TREATING BABY'S SKIN PROBLEMS

Even with the best of care, your baby's delicate skin is still susceptible to certain skin conditions. Some can be quite uncomfortable, and some may require your pediatrician's attention. But with a little know-how you can safely treat many common skin problems at home.

Diaper Rash

As long as you have your infant in diapers, there is a good chance that she will get diaper rash at least once. The cause: a wet diaper holds urine next to the skin. Prolonged contact results in irritation, and angry red patches with tiny pimples flare up. Bacteria in the feces can make a case of diaper rash even worse. Below are some simple strategies that can help to prevent an outbreak of diaper rash.

PREVENTING DIAPER RASH

- Your best defense against diaper rash is to change diapers frequently—about ten to twelve times a day is normal.
- Each time you change a diaper, be careful to remove every trace of feces by gently cleansing the skin and wiping it from front to back with a clean, damp washcloth.
- Rinse skin thoroughly and blot dry—rubbing will only irritate the skin further. Smooth on a protective diaper rash ointment. (Have your pediatrician recommend one.)
- Opt for cloth diapers rather than disposables, which have plastic covers, and try not to use rubber or plastic pants. Plastic and rubber seem to lock in moisture and trap body heat, which can inflame and irritate the skin.
- If using cloth diapers is not practical for you, try this tip from Frances Storrs, M.D., professor of dermatology at Oregon Health Sciences University: Take the plastic off the disposable diaper—it is the plastic that "bandages in" the irritants that cause diaper rash. After fastening the disposable diaper, put a regular cloth diaper over it. This double-diapering method provides extra absorbency without sealing in irritants.
- Make sure that diapers are clean and soft to the touch. Scratchy diapers can chafe tender skin. Diapers made of 100 percent cotton feel especially comfortable next to baby's skin. But cloth diapers made with blends of nylon, polyester, or other synthetics are more absorbent and waterproof.
- When laundering cloth diapers opt for a dermatologist-tested laundry detergent. These formulas are free of perfumes and dyes, which can irritate tender skin. And choose liquid fabric softeners meant to be used in the rinse rather than the scented paper squares that are tossed in the dryer. Just be sure to rinse out the fabric softener completely. Diaper services rinse cloth diapers in a germ-resistant solution. While using a diaper service costs more than laundering your diapers at home, it saves time. Besides, it is less expensive and may be

more environmentally friendly than using some types of disposable diapers.

TREATING DIAPER RASH

- If your baby does get an outbreak of diaper rash, always cleanse and rinse the diaper area thoroughly. You may want to use mildly warm tap water instead of a cleanser, as there is less risk of further irritating baby's skin. Make sure skin is completely dry before putting on a fresh diaper.
- Step up the frequency of changing diapers. If a bad case of diaper rash is keeping your infant awake, you may need to change her diaper during the night.
- Smooth on a diaper rash ointment with zinc oxide as recommended by your pediatrician. Two choices include Desitin and Johnson's Baby Diaper Rash Relief. This acts as a barrier between wetness from the diaper and baby's skin. The ointment also speeds up healing.
- On warm days let your baby go bare-bottomed whenever possible. The less contact with a wet diaper, the better!

If Diaper Rash Doesn't Clear Up

If baby's diaper rash doesn't start to improve after a few days of following the above steps, you may need to call your pediatrician. Certain bacteria and yeast thrive in warm, moist environments, which can lead to a yeast infection in the area irritated by diaper rash. Signs of this secondary infection: small pimples with whiteheads, called satellite pustules, near the diaper rash area, and blisters.

You can treat a yeast infection with a hydrocortisone cream and an antifungal cream such as Lotrimin, both of which are available over the counter. You should also continue to use your diaper rash ointment or a zinc oxide paste as part of baby's diapering routine. If a few days of at-home treatment don't do the trick, a trip to your pediatrician's office is a must!

Do keep in mind that it is quite possible for your baby to be allergic to a particular substance or skin care product that touches the diaper area. Potential irritants include detergents, fabric softeners, fragrances, alcohol, lanolin, lotions, powders, disposable diapers, and rubber pants. If you suspect that your baby is sensitive to any of the above, consult a pediatric dermatologist.

Newborn Acne

We think of a newborn baby's skin as velvety smooth, irresistibly sweet smelling, and blemish-free. So if your infant breaks out with what looks like acne, you're likely to be concerned. Relax! Your baby simply has a case of newborn acne, which is quite common and no cause for alarm.

Within three to six weeks after birth, some babies develop blackheads and whiteheads (pimples with white centers) on and around the nose. These mild acne flare-ups can also appear on the back and near the scalp.

Newborn acne—the medical term is *neonatal acne*—is thought to result when the mother's hormones stimulate the oil glands of the fetus during pregnancy. The good news is that in most cases it either improves greatly or disappears within a few weeks without special treatment. To care for newborn acne:

- Do keep your baby's skin clean. Gentle cleansing with a mild, unscented baby soap and warm water on a clean, soft, damp washcloth is all it takes.
- Do not rub—this can further irritate newborn acne.
- If your baby's skin doesn't show signs of improving after a few days of treatment, you may want to see your pediatrician.
- Some doctors may suggest treating a persistent condition with a mild 2½ percent benzoyl peroxide solution, available at drugstores. If you follow this suggestion, apply the solution sparingly. Benzoyl peroxide can be drying to baby's skin in some cases.

Beyond the newborn period, your child may develop *infantile acne*, which has been known to last as long as eighteen months. When a case of infantile acne is severe, pustules (tiny white pus-filled pimples and blisters) can develop. In such cases, topical antibiotics may be prescribed. If a case of infantile acne persists despite treatment, your doctor may prescribe erythromycin, to be taken orally.

Cradle Cap

Does your infant appear to have dandruff? What looks like an oily, dandrufflike buildup on an infant's head is *seborrhea*, which is quite harmless. Referred to as cradle cap, this condition gets its name from the accumulation of grease and dead, yellowish scales that coat baby's scalp like a cap.

Among infants cradle cap is common, but children up to six years of age can also be susceptible to seborrhea. The cause has not been determined, but it is not a serious skin condition and often clears up in a few months. Left unchecked, however, it can spread to other areas of the body including the forehead, eyebrows, behind baby's ears, and in the folds of the diaper area.

CONTROLLING CRADLE CAP

- To loosen the scales and wash away the oily coating, gently shampoo your baby's hair and scalp daily, using a mild, unscented baby soap, water, and a clean, soft washcloth.
- For stubborn cases massage a small amount of baby oil into the scalp. The oil acts as a lubricant to soften the dead scales and crusty patches.
- Next, cover the scalp with a warm towel to speed up the softening process. After fifteen minutes, gently loosen scales with a fine-tooth comb and wash them away.
- Use your comb with a light hand. Pulling out any hairs with the scales is painful for your baby and may cause temporary hair loss.
- Children with cradle cap are vulnerable to skin infection. If cradle cap resists treatment after several weeks of at-home care, seek professional help.

Prickly Heat

When the weather turns hot and humid, you may notice tiny red bumps in the creases of baby's skin, especially in the folds of the neck, shoulders, and upper chest. This condition, called prickly heat or heat rash, occurs when the pores leading to the sweat glands are blocked. The blocked sweat inflames the skin. To soothe prickly heat, follow this easy step-by-step plan.

COOL RELIEF FOR PRICKLY HEAT

- Bathe your baby frequently with cool water to calm inflammation.
- Keep your baby's skin cool and dry. You may want to smooth on a little baby powder to help absorb the excess moisture that can aggravate prickly heat.
- Dress your baby in light, loose-fitting clothes to keep her from becoming overheated. (Tight garments trap body heat and chafe the skin.) Natural fibers such as cotton are best because they allow air to circulate.
- Use a fan or air conditioner to keep baby's surroundings cool and comfortable.
- Go easy with baby oil and/or oil-rich baby lotions. Any oily film on baby's skin can block the pores. You may want to discontinue use until the rash clears up.
- Check for blisters. If any appear on the bumps, consult your pediatrician. And if prickly heat shows little sign of improving after a few days or becomes severe, visit your pediatrician.

Eczema

If you or your spouse (or a close relative) has ever had eczema—a dry, itchy, scaly rash with blisters—chances are that your baby may have inherited a predisposition to develop this skin condition. Doctors are unsure of what exactly causes an outbreak of eczema. Sources that can trigger a flare-up in a predisposed child include dry indoor heating (lack of humidity dehydrates the skin) and allergic reactions to a substance that touches the skin or to a food.

Your baby can break out with her first case of eczema at a few months of age or later on during the toddler stage (one to two years of age). With careful treatment, a mild case of eczema should clear up.

SOOTHING SKIN CARE FOR ECZEMA

- To relieve itching apply a prescription or nonprescription hydrocortisone ointment.
- Bathe your child with mildly warm water and a gentle soap. Superfatted soaps won't dry out baby's skin. Oatmeal-based soaps are also mild and are formulated to relieve itching.
- Do not overbathe your baby. Cleansing more than a few times a week can strip the skin of protective oils. Be sure to rinse off every trace of soap.
- Keep your baby's fingernails clipped short. If tiny nails scratch eczema, the blisters may break open. When the ooze dries, it worsens the itching.
- Use a humidifier or vaporizer to add moisture to the air.

If the rash looks as if it is becoming infected—signs include inflammation, swelling, and tenderness—call your pediatrician immediately. You should also see your doctor if a week of at-home treatment doesn't help. Questions regarding your baby's diet should also be addressed to a doctor.

Impetigo

If your child is exposed to someone who has impetigo, he can "catch" this condition. Impetigo is a bacterial infection of the skin, and it is especially contagious among infants. (Older children are also susceptible to impetigo.) Clusters of soft, yellowish, fluid-filled blisters appear on the surface of the skin. When a blister breaks it oozes a brownish yellow fluid and leaves a flat, reddish area.

Although it is not a serious skin condition, impetigo can spread quickly from one part of the body to another, and to other children and adults upon contact with the skin of an infected individual. If you act quickly, impetigo clears up with proper treatment. Simply follow these steps based on recommendations from the American Academy of Dermatology.

R$_x$ FOR IMPETIGO

- Gently cleanse the skin two or three times a day with a mild soap and warm water.
- If washing isn't enough to soften the crusts, try loosening them with warm compresses. As the crust softens, use a light touch to rub away crusts and pus.
- Massage a topical antibiotic over sores at least three times a day. Continue to apply antibiotic cream three or four times a day until all scabs are removed.
- Keep your child's nails short. Scratching spreads the infection to other parts of the body.
- To help minimize the spread of infection to other family members, make sure they don't share personal items that touch the skin, such as washcloths and bath towels.
- Be on the lookout for symptoms of impetigo in other family members.
- If home treatment doesn't keep impetigo in check or fails to improve the condition, see your pediatrician.

COMING CLEAN: THE SCOOP ON SOAP

By the time your child is ready to graduate from baby soap, you may want to switch to the same soap that you buy for the rest of your family. Not any soap will do, however. For example, a strong deodorant soap is fine for adolescents and adults who have a problem with body odor, but it may be too harsh for a child's sensitive skin.

Deodorant soaps leave antibacterial agents such as *triclocarban* and *triclosan* on the skin. These ingredients kill the bacteria that cause body odor, but they may also irritate tender skin. (And since there are no odor-producing sweat glands on the face, there is no point in washing the face with a deodorant soap.) Many are also highly fragranced.

If you yourself like to bathe and shower with a deodorant soap but want a bath soap that the whole family can share, you may want to try a deodorant soap made with moisturizers, such as Lever 2000. Read labels! Not all deodorant soaps contain moisturizing ingredients.

Gritty soaps are also a bad choice because they are too abrasive. These soaps often contain tiny grains of pumice, a lightweight volcanic glass with polishing properties. (Pumice is the same material used to make the pedicure stones that skim hard, dry skin off your feet, so you can imagine how hardworking gritty soaps are!)

What you want for your child is a soap that washes away dirt and grime without stripping the protective natural oils that keep skin moist. When these oils are repeatedly removed and skin loses moisture, the skin is easily irritated and more vulnerable to reddening and chapping.

Scoping Out Soaps

Plain soap is a mixture of animal or vegetable fats and alkali salts, ingredients that do an excellent job of cleansing but can also dry and irritate the skin. Again, check labels. If a soap lists *sodium tallowate*, *sodium cocoate*, and *sodium palm kernelate* as the only ingredients, it is highly alkaline and too strong for regular use for children.

Many dermatologists recommend *neutral soaps*, cleansing bars that are neither too alkaline nor too acidic. Often referred to as soapless soaps or soap-free soaps, neutral soaps are made with gentle synthetic detergents. (Don't let the word *detergent* scare you—cleansing bars formulated with synthetic detergents are made to be less alkaline, less drying, and less irritating than plain soap.)

Mild synthetic cleansers listed on labels include *sodium cocoyl isethionate* and *sodium isethionate*. Among the mildest neutral soaps are *superfatted* formulas such as Basis. Fats such as *stearic acid* or *coconut acid* are added to *neutralize* any alkali in the formula.

One soap that rates a gold star for gentleness from many dermatologists is Dove, which is not a soap at all but a neutral superfatted cleansing bar made with one-quarter moisturizing cream. Because it was developed for sensitive or allergic skin, Dove is recommended as safe for children.

More Skin-soothing Ingredients

Of course, there's more than one neutral soap trusted by dermatologists that does a thorough job of cleansing, yet is mild enough for children. The following is a checklist of some of the key ingredients that are kind to skin.

Colloidal oatmeal is produced by dry-milling the edible part of whole oat kernels into a fine talclike powder. The anti-itch properties of colloidal oatmeal help to bring relief to such skin irritations as diaper rash, eczema, chicken pox, sunburn, poison ivy, and other skin allergies. Aveeno makes a gentle soap with colloidal oatmeal.

Dextrin is an ingredient similar to cornstarch. Like cornstarch, it helps to calm irritated skin. A cleansing bar with dextrin, such as Lowila, is ideal for children with eczema or other skin allergies.

Glycerine is a humectant, an ingredient that attracts and binds moisture to the skin. Transparent cleansing bars such as Neutrogena and Pears Soap are made with glycerine. *Note:* Avoid glycerine soaps formulated for *oily skin.* They contain oil-blotting astringents, which are too drying for young skin.

Lanolin, an oil derived from the wool of sheep, is an excellent moisturizer. While cleansing bars with this skin-softening ingredient are mild, some allergy-prone individuals may have an adverse reaction to lanolin.

Plant extracts include aloe vera, chamomile, licorice root, kola nut extract, and wild pansy among others. Plant extracts used in soap and other skin care products relieve itching and reduce inflammation.

STEP-BY-STEP FACE CLEANSING

By the time children are old enough to begin to brush their teeth (around age two), they may also be ready to learn how to wash up. Be prepared for lots of splashing! With a toddler or preschooler, of course, you will have to do most of the work. Young children who aren't tall enough to reach the sink may need a step stool. Then again, it may be easier if your child can lather up in the tub during his bath.

If you have an older child who does a hit-or-miss job of face washing, you can give him a refresher course. After all, it's never too late to learn the good skin care habits that lead to a lifetime of clear, glowing skin. The following steps will make it easy.

1. Fill the washbasin (or tub) with mildly warm water. Have your child gently splash her face with water and wet the cleansing bar. (If you opt for a gentle liquid cleanser, pour a small amount into your child's hands.)
2. Have your child work up a lather in the palms of her hands. Using fingertips, massage the foam into her skin with circular strokes. (Or use a *clean, soft* washcloth.)
3. Show your child how to massage the soap or cleanser from cheeks to chin, then from nose to forehead, gliding fingers from the center of the face out toward the hairline.
4. Whether your child uses her fingertips or a washcloth, make sure she does not scrub! Rubbing can irritate and redden the skin.
5. Do not massage lather into the skin for more than fifteen seconds. Soap or cleanser left on the skin longer than that can dry and irritate skin.
6. Make sure your child rinses well with at least eight to ten splashes of clear lukewarm water. Again, any soapy film left on the skin can be drying.
7. Show your child how to blot her face well with a soft, clean towel. Remember, no brisk rubbing. The less skin is handled, the better.

Your child shouldn't have to wash his face with soap and water (or cleanser) more than once or twice a day. Cleansing can be part of his bedtime ritual. In the morning, splashing the face with clear lukewarm water is enough.

What if you can't get near your child with soap and water or a washcloth? An editor at *Parents* magazine tells me that her three-year-old son prefers cleaning his face with a baby wipe or cleansing towelette. Either one does the trick to clean up chocolate icing or spaghetti sauce in a pinch!

HINTS FOR HAND WASHING

Keeping a child's busy hands clean is not always easy. You may, however, want your child to step up hand washing during the cold and flu season. There is medical evidence that one virus that causes sneezes and sniffles contaminates the *hands* of people who catch colds.

When a healthy person touches the hand of a cold sufferer or a contaminated article, the cold virus spreads to the healthy person's hands. Scratching the nose or rubbing the eyes with contaminated hands can be all it takes to become infected with a cold.

Through hand contact a chain of contamination is set in motion, passing on the virus from cold victim to healthy individual. It doesn't require much to imagine what can happen if a few children in a daycare center come down with colds! In fact, studies show that preschoolers catch cold twice as often as adults.

To make hand washing a habit you may want to keep a liquid cleanser in a handy pump bottle by your kitchen and bathroom sinks. (Pumps are fun to use and easier to manage than a slippery bar of soap.) Be sure that the formula contains emollient ingredients such as lanolin to prevent chapping and to keep skin soft. Today antibacterial liquid formulas such as Liquid Dial are also available with moisturizing ingredients. Whatever product you choose, make sure that your child follows these easy steps:

1. Wash hands with soap or cleanser and warm—not hot—running water.

Skin Deep

2. Don't be hit-or-miss. Wash backs of hands as well as palms, and don't forget fingernails.
3. Rinse well and gently blot hands with a clean towel or fresh paper towel.
4. Teach your child to turn off the faucet with a paper towel when at school or in a public restroom. This minimizes the risk of picking up cold germs from a contaminated faucet.

REMEDY FOR CHAPPED HANDS

When your child comes in from the cold with chapped hands, try this soothing treatment from skin care expert and busy mother Lia Schorr of Lia Schorr Skin Care Salon, New York City, author of the book *Lia Schorr's Seasonal Skin Care:* Soak your child's hands in mildly warm water for a minute or two. Gently pat hands dry with a towel. Next, massage a dab of petroleum jelly into hands and fingers, or use a few drops of baby oil. Allow it to absorb into the skin. Reapply another thin layer of petroleum jelly or baby oil. If your child's hands are especially raw and red, you may want to apply an over-the-counter hydrocortisone cream or ointment. (Ask your pediatrician.) Apply it to your child's hands, then smooth on a fragrance-free hand cream or lotion to lock in the skin's natural oils.

When your child needs to wash his hands, have him try a soap-free dermatologist-tested creamy cleanser. Smooth it over hands and fingers, then tissue it off. Or try a nonalkaline cleansing bar made with moisturizing cream.

An ounce of prevention can help to minimize the chances of chapping. Before your child goes outdoors into the cold weather, rub a little hand cream or lotion onto your child's hands. Then slip on her mittens or gloves.

BODY LOTIONS

Once out of diapers, does your child need a body lotion on a regular basis? Not really. Body lotions are not necessary for youngsters unless dry skin is a problem, according to Amy Paller, M.D., associate professor of pediatrics and dermatology at Northwestern University and head of the division of dermatology at Children's Memorial Hospital, Chicago. If your child's skin is mildly dry, Dr. Paller suggests using a light, water-based lotion. (*Hint:* The first ingredient listed on the label is *water.*) If your child's skin is extremely dry (flaky and itchy), use a water-in-oil cream, which is richer in skin-softening emollients than a water-based lotion. (Your child is more likely to need a rich cream when the weather turns cold and skin loses more moisture.) Whatever product you choose, apply it sparingly and only as needed.

ARE HYPOALLERGENIC PRODUCTS SAFE?

Many products formulated for children are labeled "hypoallergenic." This means that the product is fragrance free and does not contain other known potential irritants and allergens. The accent is on *known*.

Sensitivity to an ingredient depends on the individual. Chances are that for most children, hypoallergenic skin care products will not cause a reaction. However, no product, no matter how "pure" it is, can be guaranteed 100 percent safe all of the time for every single person who uses it. If you suspect that any product is irritating your child's skin, toss it. Allergic reactions should be checked by your child's doctor.

TIPS FOR CHAPPED LIPS

Raw, chapped lips can be painful for a child. Wind, cold, and low humidity rob lips of the moisture they need to keep the delicate tissues soft and smooth. As the outer layers of the skin dry out, lips become rough and cracked. To treat and prevent chapped lips, follow this easy plan.

- Try to discourage your child from licking her lips to soften dry, chapped skin. It only makes the problem worse! As the saliva evaporates, lips lose more moisture.
- Apply a protective lip balm or ointment to your child's lips before she goes outdoors. Young children love mint- and

fruit-flavored lip balm sticks. A *light* coating of petroleum jelly also works in a pinch. Protection is also needed indoors—dry, heated air also saps moisture from lips.
- A quick slick of lip balm or ointment at bedtime will also soothe lips while your child sleeps—and won't come off on his pillow.
- If you're planning a family ski trip, take along lip care products with sunscreen. At high altitudes you're closer to the sun, and a high percentage of sunlight bounces off snow. Unprotected lips burn easily and need a product to filter out the sun's harmful rays.

TREATING A COLD SORE

If your child has ever gotten cold sores, you know how nasty they can be. Cold sores or fever blisters are tiny blisters. They can appear as clusters or singly, and show up on or near the lips, such as the corner of the mouth. Cold sores can also develop on the nose, chin, or cheeks. They are caused by the Herpes Simplex Virus (HSV) Type I—not HSV Type II, which usually affects the genital area after sexual contact with a person infected with the virus.

First-time infections with cold sores often occur during childhood, and recurrent flare-ups are usually mild. Children catch this virus via kissing or by being physically close (hugging, rubbing noses) to a family member, relative, or friend who is infected. A cold, fever, or overexposure to sunlight can cause an outbreak.

The itching and burning of a cold sore can be quite painful for a child. You can try to relieve a cold sore with a medicated lip salve or lip ointment formulated to treat cold sores. Common healing ingredients are camphor and phenol. Or you can try one of these simple home remedies.

- Apply a compress of cold salt water. Add one teaspoon of salt to one pint of cold water. Apply a clean washcloth soaked in this solution for ten to fifteen minutes several times a day.
- Brew a cup of plain tea such as Lipton's. Allow it to cool until mildly warm, then apply the wet tea bag to the cold

sore for several minutes. Reapply as needed. It is the tannic acid in the tea that soothes the pain.
- Dab on a light coating of petroleum jelly with a cotton swab. The petroleum jelly helps to protect the cold sore against abrasion.
- To speed up drying of a cold sore, apply witch hazel with a piece of fresh sterile cotton. Witch hazel also has natural disinfectant properties.

If the cold sore doesn't clear up quickly or your child has recurring painful outbreaks, a doctor's prescription may be necessary. Consult your pediatrician. An infant with a cold sore should be taken to the doctor right away.

NAIL CARE FOR KIDS

You want your child to be well groomed right down to her fingertips and toes. Of course, there's more to nail care than improving your child's appearance. Ragged nails can catch on clothing (or Mom's pantyhose) and then split or break off, which can hurt.

Keeping nails clean and trim will help to prevent certain hand and foot problems, such as painful hangnails and ingrown toenails. And curing bad habits such as picking at cuticles and nail biting can also prevent infections.

Your Baby's Nails

You want to keep your baby's nails short and smooth to keep her from scratching herself—and you. Because tiny fingernails grow quickly, you may have to trim her nails twice a week. An infant's toenails don't grow as quickly, so you won't have to trim them as often. Once or twice a month is plenty. Some babies may not need to have their toenails clipped for the first six months.

The best time to trim your baby's nails: after a bath, when the water has softened her nails. However, if your baby fusses or fidgets, wait until she's asleep. Here are a few of the nail care supplies to keep on hand.

- Safety baby scissors with blunt tips or child-size nail clippers. (Revlon Care for Kids makes baby manicure implements.)
- A buffing disc or a nail shaper (a smooth emery board) for smoothing rough edges of nails. A fine-textured emery board made for soft nails is another option.
- Rubbing alcohol and fresh sterile cotton or alcohol pads for sanitizing clippers and scissors. Wipe implements clean before and after each use.

Whether you opt for scissors or clippers, trim fingernails straight across, at the top of baby's fingertips. Toenails should also be clipped straight across using a nail clipper—scissors may nick the skin. To smooth any rough edges, take your buffing disc or nail shaper. Hold it at a slight angle to your child's nail. Lightly stroke the nail from the corner to the center in one direction only. *Do not saw back and forth!* It's too rough on delicate nails. And do not file too deeply into the corners. This makes nails more vulnerable to tears and splits. Repeat on the opposite side. The small, soft nails of babies (and of small children) can be smoothed in a few light, quick strokes.

Be on the lookout for ingrown toenails, nails that turn under and grow into the skin. Babies' nails are so soft that they may appear to be ingrown. Usually this is nothing to worry about, but if the skin around the toenail or fingernail becomes inflamed or tender, call your pediatrician.

Nail Care for Toddlers and Up

As your child grows, his baby-soft nails will become harder. Luckily, nail care for kids is a low-maintenance task. A soak in the tub is enough to help nails come clean. Stubborn grime can be loosened with a light scrubbing using a nail brush and a mild soap. Child-size brushes in colorful animal shapes such as ducks and hedgehogs can make a simple chore more fun. Be sure the bristles are soft. And once the bristles become worn out, toss the brush. Frayed bristles can scratch.

A weekly trim after your child's bath should be enough to keep fingernails and toenails neat. Follow the same steps described for baby's nail care (above). Reminder: cut toenails straight across to prevent ingrown toenails. If you curve the nail too deeply at the corners or clip them too short, the nail can grow into the skin. (Nails need to reach the tip of the toe to cushion the skin against rubbing and pressure from shoes and socks.)

By the time your child is around ten, she can begin to take on more responsibility for her nail care. To help prevent dry, ragged cuticles, show your child how to rub a lotion into nails and cuticles after a bath. When cuticles are soft and neat, it helps your child to resist the urge to pick at them.

Boys in particular may find these nail care steps unappealing; in this case it helps if Dad follows his own nail-grooming routine. This way your son can see that having clean, trim nails and cuticles is also important for men. For both boys and girls alike, you may want to invest in a nail care kit that includes a nail brush, fine-grain emery boards, and hand lotion. Having a set of nail grooming basics that is theirs alone may step up enthusiasm for nail care.

Help for Hangnails

A hangnail hurts. It is a split or tear in the skin along the side or base of the fingernail. One cause is dryness. With excess water loss, the skin becomes less elastic and may crack. If your child has a habit of picking the skin and cuticle around the nail, he can also get a hangnail. An injury such as a paper cut is another common cause. If your child is prone to getting hangnails, be sure to rub a good hand cream or lotion into his hands, nails, and cuticles a few times a day. Moisturized skin is less likely to split.

To treat a hangnail, carefully snip the tip of dry skin with sterile manicure scissors. Do not attempt to peel off the hangnail! Pulling it off will injure the skin around it. Dab the area with an antiseptic lotion such as Sea Breeze. This will help to prevent an infection. What if the hangnail becomes inflamed or looks infected or if pus forms? Call your pediatrician. Your child may need medication.

Breaking the Nail-biting Habit

About the time your child has given up on thumb sucking (around age three), she may move on to nail biting. Nibbling on nails gives many children a quiet way to console themselves when they feel anxious. Unfortunately this nervous quirk can persist into the teen years and beyond. Stubby, ragged nails do nothing for your child's appearance. And once he starts to care about his looks, there may be times when he wants to make a good impression but hides his hands out of embarrassment.

However, nail biting can do more damage than puncturing your child's self-esteem. Gnawing on nails can cause painful hangnails. It can cause an infection around the nail called *paronychia*. If your child picks at his cuticles, he is also susceptible to this infection.

Nibbling nails and cuticles damages the skin's natural barrier against infection. Signs of infection under and around the nail bed are inflammation, tenderness, and swelling; pus may also form. Eventually the nail plate may develop white horizontal ridges.

If your child has a habit of gnawing on his nails, be sure to check his hands on a regular basis. If it looks as if an infection has flared up, take him to the doctor. In most cases the infection will be treated with an antifungal ointment or topical antibiotic. Or your child may need to take an oral antibiotic.

To allow the infection to heal you also need to help your child put a halt to the habit of nail biting. This is not easy, especially if your child chews his nails as a way to dispel anxiety. You may want to consult your pediatrician on this score. In the meantime, take steps to keep your child's nails clean and trim. The better his nails look, the less tempted your child may be to bite them off.

Apply a coat of clear polish to nails. (Bitten nails are weak and prone to peeling; the polish adds a layer of protection.) If your son thinks that glossy clear polish makes him look like a sissy, opt for a clear polish or base coat with a nonshiny matte finish. If all else fails, you can always try to coat your child's nails with a bitter-tasting polish from the drugstore. Theory has it that the polish tastes so bad that it will help your child resist the urge to bite. There are no guarantees, but it's worth a try!

With preteens, you may be able to appeal to their desire to look more attractive. Ask your child to imagine how good he can look and how much better he would feel if he didn't bite his nails. Practice a little behavior modification. When he's tempted to gnaw on his nails, suggest that he close his eyes, take a deep breath, and count to ten as he slowly exhales. This should help to relieve anxiety better than biting his nails. And you can always try the reward system. For every week that your child doesn't bite his nails, give him a small treat.

In time, finding healthier ways to cope with tension and taking pride in personal appearance should help to kick this nervous habit.

FIRST-RATE FIRST AID FOR CUTS AND SCRAPES

My mother is a registered nurse, and as my six brothers and sisters and I were growing up, she was always on call to rescue us with her medical expertise. Falls from bicycles and slips on roller skates were among our nonstop emergencies.

There were times, of course, when we needed stitches or a doctor's attention. But our mother's knowledge of basic first aid kept things under control until we got to the doctor's office or hospital emergency room. You don't, of course, have to be a nurse to mend most cuts and scrapes. They are easy to treat and heal quickly. By learning a few simple first-aid skills you can cope with these minor injuries.

R_x FOR CUTS AND SCRAPES

- To prevent infecton, cleanse the affected area with an antibacterial soap and water. With a baby or toddler, this may be easier to manage by putting your child into a tepid bath and gently washing the cut with a clean, soapy washcloth. For older children, cuts on arms and legs can be rinsed clean with running water; however, cuts on the head, face, and torso should be cleansed with a clean washcloth and soap to remove dirt and bacteria.
- To stop bleeding, apply direct pressure with a spotlessly clean handkerchief or washcloth for five to ten minutes. Do not use cotton balls, as tiny fibers can settle into the cut. Resist the temptation to peek at the cut before five minutes are up—bleeding can start up again. If bleeding doesn't stop after applying pressure for ten minutes, call your doctor.

- Applying an antibacterial ointment is optional. You may want to apply an adhesive-strip bandgage to keep out dirt and debris, but it is not essential. *Note:* An infant may want to chew on her bandage and could choke. When treating a baby, you may want to skip using adhesive bandages altogether.
- If you think that any foreign matter such as glass or dirt may be trapped in the wound, see your doctor. A small child in pain is not likely to tolerate your own attempts to look for dirt and debris. Your pediatrician will use a local anesthetic to numb the pain before examining your child's injury.
- As your child's cut heals, be on the alert for redness, swelling, or pus. Call your doctor immediately if these signs of infection show up. You should also call your doctor if bleeding recurs.

THE BEST BANDAGES

Bandages printed with colorful cartoon characters are a big hit with the preschool set. Kids are less apt to peel off their bandages if they sport a beloved hero or heroine. Kids also love the dazzling colors of Day-Glo bandages.

For a better fit, choose kid-sized bandages. Along with standard plastic adhesive bandages, you should also be able to find stretchy fabric strips. Their flexibility adds to their staying power. There are also special shapes designed for hard-to-fit places such as knuckles, elbows, and knees. To make sure the bandage is "ouchless," look for those with absorbent nonstick pads. They are less likely to irritate the cut and won't stick when it's time to take off the bandage.

Does Your Child Need Stitches?

Be aware that a deep gash, especially if it is on your child's face and/or scalp, may need stitches. Even if the wound does not look serious or doesn't bleed much, you should call your doctor immediately. A deep wound can do serious damage to the nerves and tendons beneath the surface of the skin. Scarring can also result from any long cut or any deep cuts on the face, chest, and back. A stitch in time can make scars less obvious. Three signals that stitches may be needed:

1. The wound has a jagged edge.
2. The wound is more than half an inch wide.
3. The wound is deep enough for flesh to protrude from it.

Be sure to check your child thoroughly from head to toe. If your child's cut does require stitches, or if you're unsure about whether he really needs stitches, call your doctor as soon as possible—within eight to twelve hours of the accident. Prompt action can minimize unsightly scarring.

Until you can get to the doctor or hospital, flush the wound with running water and apply direct pressure as described above. In an emergency, a clean cotton cloth doubles as a bandage.

MAKEUP AND MASKS

Around the age of three or four, many little girls and boys begin to play with Mommy's makeup. However, the pigments, chemical ingredients, and preservatives used in makeup formulated for adults make your cosmetics too strong for young skin. Your eye makeup is especially hazardous. Eye makeup, especially mascara and liquid eyeliner, spoils quickly. And if contaminated mascara or eyeliner comes into contact with a scratched cornea, an eye infection may result.

But you don't have to spoil your child's fun or squelch his or her creativity. If your son or daughter likes to play dress-up with makeup, look into makeup especially formulated for children such as the Barbie and Little Mermaid collections. These child-friendly makeup kits usually consist of a sheer lip gloss, a talc face powder with a hint of blush, and a water-based peel-off nail polish.

I have a young friend, Kira, now eleven years old, who loves to slather on her mom's facial masks. However, facial masks made for adults are too strong for young skin. Many have ingredients meant to draw out oil or to skim off dry, flaky skin. If your child insists on indulging in a face mask, whip up this easy skin-safe version. (Kira's mom was thrilled with this recipe!)

- Mix a half-cup (or less) of plain yogurt with a teaspoon of honey. Yogurt and honey help to work up a glow by accelerating the blood supply to the skin. This soothing mixture stays creamy and won't harden.
- Apply to the face and allow the mixture to set for five minutes. Rinse off with fresh cotton soaked with lukewarm water. (Many skin care experts believe that fresh cotton is more hygienic and less irritating than a washcloth.)
- Once the yogurt and honey mixture is rinsed off, splash face with cool water. Pat skin dry and apply a *thin* layer of a gentle vitamin E-enriched cream to the face.

By following the simple skin care strategies in this chapter, your child should grow up with beautiful skin that blooms with rosy good health. Should any problems or questions concerning your child's skin care arise, always consult your child's doctor. You may also want to see a pediatric dermatologist, a skin doctor who specializes in the care and treatment of children.

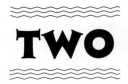

TWO

Rub-a-Dub-Dub: Tips for the Tub

BATHING BASICS ARE part of everyday skin care and go a long way toward keeping your child's skin velvety smooth and glowing with good health. Most young children love to splash in the tub with their bath toys. But occasionally you may have to negotiate with a bath-shy child who has to be coaxed into the tub. And then, by the time your child hits the preteen years, you'll be banging on the bathroom door, demanding that he give you equal time in the shower!

This chapter will tell you how to make bath time safe, simple, and bubbling up with fun. For the newborn, there is a step-by-step plan for gentle sponge-bathing as well as tips for her first tub bath. And to add to baby's bath-time pleasure, there is a soothing massage to relax and comfort her. For children of all ages there are guidelines on bath and shower safety—how to prevent slips, how to protect your child against scalding from hot water, and more. You'll also learn how to choose and use the best bubble bath products and how to whip up your own skin-smoothing bath treats with ingredients from your kitchen. There are surefire strategies to get a reluctant tot into the tub. And tips on introducing your child to the shower, plus notes on your growing child's need for privacy in the bathroom. When you think of all the time your child will spend enjoying this indoor water sport, you'll want to do whatever you can to make bath and shower time safe and happy.

BATHING YOUR BABY

The soothing strokes and splashes of bathing your baby make bath time a pleasant ritual for both parent and child. Gently soaping your baby's body, wrapping her up in a cozy towel afterward, and holding her close to breathe in the sweetness of her skin—it's no wonder you look forward to your baby's bath!

To keep your infant's skin clean and soft, you do not need to bathe her every day—in fact, overbathing is one of the leading causes of dry, flaky, and/or itchy skin. Two or three baths a week are sufficient during baby's first year, as long as the face and genital area are kept clean. Many pediatricians also advise that you only sponge-bathe your baby until the remnant of the umbilical cord falls off and the navel is fully healed.

Easy-does-it Sponge Bath

To gently sponge-bathe your baby you will need:

- A mild, unscented soap
- A soft washcloth
- Sterile cotton balls
- Cotton swabs
- Rubbing alcohol
- A bowl of warm water

1. Because it is important to keep your baby warm, you can keep her dressed in her undershirt and diaper during her sponge bath. Place her on the changing table or on the sponge cushion that comes with a portable baby tub.
2. Dip a sterile cotton ball into plain warm water and gently wipe one eye, starting at the inner corner. Take a fresh cotton ball to cleanse the other eye. Next, use another cotton ball and warm water to wash around and behind baby's

ears. Last, using either fresh cotton or a damp washcloth, wash around baby's mouth, chin, and neck with warm water only.
3. Tuck your baby against your upper body, and as you cradle her head in your hand and support her neck and back with your arm, hold her above a bowl of warm water. Wet her scalp; using the pads of your fingertips, massage a little baby soap into her scalp. Rinse off the soap and pat baby's head dry. *Note:* To keep soap out of baby's eyes, you may want to rinse her head with a wet washcloth.
4. Take off your baby's undershirt. (If she doesn't like being naked, try uncovering and cleansing one area at a time.) Using a damp washcloth and baby soap, cleanse baby's arms, chest, and neck. Be sure to get into the folds and creases of her skin. As you cleanse baby's hands, check for any traces of lint between fingers. Rinse off soap with mildly warm water and pat skin dry.
5. Next, support your baby's head in your hand and carefully turn her on her side. Gently soap and rinse baby's back. After patting skin dry, slip on baby's undershirt.
6. Soak a cotton swab in rubbing alcohol. With a light touch, swab baby's navel down to the base. *Do not wet* the navel area until the navel has fully healed.
7. Next, take off baby's diaper and cleanse the genitals, buttocks, legs, and feet. Rinse off soap and pat baby's skin dry. If your baby has diaper rash, smooth on an ointment as approved by your doctor. Put on a fresh diaper and clothe your baby.

INTO THE TUB!

Once baby's umbilical cord has fallen off and the navel area has completely healed, he may be ready for his first tub bath. We say "may" because there is a chance that he won't like being immersed in water at first. Be patient. You can continue to sponge-bathe your baby for a while. Eventually he will love the splish-splash of a tub bath!

Baby-tub Bath

To make tub time fun and safe for baby, follow this easy step-by-step plan. You will need:

- A portable plastic baby tub with a nonskid bottom and a slip-proof sponge cushion
- Unscented baby soap or cleanser
- A soft washcloth
- A no-tears baby shampoo

1. Place your baby tub on a sturdy table or countertop. Either surface should be at a height that's comfortable for you. Make sure the room is comfortably warm and draft-free.
2. To control the water temperature, run cold water into the tub first; gradually add hot water until it feels pleasantly warm. (Two inches of water is plenty!) To test the water, immerse the inside of your wrist.
3. To ease your baby into the tub, slip one hand under his bottom, then cradle his head and neck with the other. To dispel any anxiety, smile and talk to your baby as you gently lower him into the tub, bottom first.
4. As you support your baby's head and neck with one arm, use a soft washcloth and baby soap or cleanser to wash his face, arms, and neck. Be sure to cleanse the folds of skin under baby's chin.
5. Tilting your baby's head downward, wet his scalp. Then shampoo his hair and scalp from front to back. These steps keep shampoo and water from getting into his eyes. Again, use the pads of your fingertips. *Note:* Don't be concerned about scrubbing the soft spot too vigorously. This area is protected with a thick membrane. Rinse away shampoo. If he has cradle cap, see page 15.
6. Next, soap your baby's tummy, arms, and legs. Look for lint between fingers, toes, and creases of skin. With the baby's back supported on the sponge cushion, lift his legs to

cleanse the genital area. Be sure to get into the folds and creases. Cleansing the genital area from front to back helps to prevent bacterial infections. Carefully rinse away soap.
7. Lift your baby into an upright position while you soap and rinse his back. Later on, when your baby is older, he can sit up without your support.
8. Be sure all traces of soap and shampoo are rinsed clean. Any soap film that clings to skin can cause irritation. Scoop your baby out of the tub with both arms and wrap him in a warm, soft towel. (A hooded towel is a good chill-chaser because it keeps body heat from escaping through baby's head.) Lightly blot his skin until he is completely dry, warm, and comfortable. After a cozy cuddle, diaper and dress your baby.

Tip: To keep bath time pleasant for both you and your child, do not bathe your baby when he is hungry or sleepy.

IMPORTANT!

Never leave your baby or toddler alone in the tub, and *never* turn your back on her. In just a few seconds a child can drown in less than two inches of water. If you must answer the door or telephone, take your baby with you.

BEFORE THE TUB, A GENTLE RUB: BABY MASSAGE

To make bath time a special delight for both you and your baby, why not give her a massage before or after her bath? A gentle massage can be a loving way to relax your baby. Just as cuddling, caressing, and rocking your baby establish an intimate connection between parent and child, a massage can be part of the everyday physical contact that brings you closer together. The tender touches of massage are also said to relieve gas and colic and to soothe tension.

Rub-a-Dub-Dub

Some experts believe that even newborn babies can be massaged, while others advise waiting until your infant is about four weeks old. Before baby's first massage, it's best to check with your pediatrician. And as long as your baby enjoys the relaxing strokes of massage, you can indulge her in these gentle rubdowns well into her first year and beyond.

MASSAGE SAFETY ALERT

There are times when you should not give your baby a massage. To play it safe, follow these guidelines.

- **Don't** massage any area of baby's skin that is red, swollen, or inflamed. Avoid any cuts.
- **Don't** massage baby's belly until the umbilical cord has fallen off and completely healed.
- **Don't** massage you baby if she has a fever. Massaging her may spread any infection present.

MASSAGE STEPS

For a safe, soothing massage, follow these easy how-tos from Diana Simkin, M.A., A.C.C.E., cofounder of Family Focus, Inc., a center for pregnancy, childbirth, and parenthood, in New York City, and coauthor with Beverly Savage of *Preparation for Birth* (Ballantine Books, 1987).

- For your baby's comfort and health, be sure to massage her in a warm, draft-free room.
- Remove any rings or bracelets that could scratch baby's delicate skin. Your fingernails should be clipped short and filed to a smooth finish. If nails are long, use pads of fingers only when massaging your baby.
- A small amount of oil will help your hands to glide smoothly over baby's skin. Opt for a natural, digestible oil such as sweet almond oil (available at health food stores).

Avoid baby oil—it is petroleum based and therefore not digestible.
- Keep a towel or diaper handy—your soothing strokes may relax the baby's bowels and bladder during massage.
- Sit comfortably. Try sitting cross-legged, with your baby cradled in your lap. Or place her on a soft pillow, blanket, or towel in front of you.
- If your doctor approves massage for a baby under four weeks old, hold your baby close to your body with one arm and massage with the other. To massage his back, hold your baby against your chest or shoulder as if to burp him. Use a featherlight touch to softly caress his skin—firmer pressure is best for older babies.
- Wait at least an hour after feeding your baby before massaging baby's tummy.
- To relax your body and clear your mind, take a few deep breaths before beginning baby's massage.
- As you apply the oil, warm it first by gently rubbing your hands together. Oil should be used sparingly. Repeat each massage stroke three times.

MASSAGING THE FACE

1. Using fingertips, softly stroke baby's forehead from the center out toward ears.
2. Using your thumbs, massage over bony arches of baby's eyebrows, stroking out toward ears.
3. Next, with index fingers or thumbs, massage under baby's eyes out to the temples. Placing index fingers on either side of nose, use long, gentle strokes to glide them across tops of cheekbones out to ears.
4. Place fingertips on each jaw joint near baby's ears. (Baby uses the muscles here when sucking or crying, and overworked muscles can become tight and tense.) Gently massage jaw with small, circular strokes. Last, massage baby's earlobes with fingertips and thumbs.

MASSAGING THE CHEST

1. Apply oil to baby's chest and shoulders. Place both hands, palms down, in the center of baby's chest. Move your hands as if you were flattening the pages of a book and glide them up toward the shoulders, then down to baby's sides. With each stroke, follow the curve of baby's rib cage.
2. Moving your hand diagonally across baby's chest, gently stroke from one side to the opposite shoulder and then back again. Repeat with the other hand on the opposite side.

MASSAGING THE BELLY

1. Smooth oil over baby's belly, then place palm or fingertips of one hand over baby's belly. Very slowly yet firmly massage baby's abdominal muscles directly around the navel area in a clockwise circle. Moving your hand in this direction follows the large intestine, helping to make elimination easier. It also helps to relieve constipation and gas.
2. Place outside of one hand to the top of baby's belly, well below the ribs. Apply pressure as your hand glides down over baby's abdomen toward tops of legs. This helps to push gas out of baby's abdomen.

MASSAGING THE LEGS AND FEET

1. Apply oil to baby's legs and feet. Holding baby's heel in one hand, encircle her thigh with fingers of opposite hand. Massage baby's leg in one smooth stroke from thigh to ankle.
2. Still holding baby's foot in one hand, encircle baby's ankle. Now massage baby's leg in one firm, gentle stroke from ankle to thigh. Next, massage baby's thighs and calves using small circular strokes.

3. Massage baby's foot from heel to toes. To massage the center of the sole, take your thumb and apply light, firm pressure using tiny circular strokes. (Massaging this sensitive spot is said to calm a crying baby.)
4. Last, open your hand and massage baby's leg in one even stroke from ankle to hip and then from hip to ankle.

MASSAGING THE BACK

1. Turn your baby over on her tummy. Smooth oil over baby's back. Using thumbs, gently knead between baby's shoulder blades with small circular strokes.
2. With fingertips spread wide apart, massage baby's back from her neck down to and over her bottom.
3. Alternating hands, stroke your hand across baby's back from shoulder to shoulder. Rest for a moment; then stroke baby's back from shoulders to buttocks, then from buttocks to shoulders.
4. Last, with open palms, massage baby up and down from toes to head, and then from head to toes.

SMALL CHILDREN AND THE BIG TUB

By the time your child has outgrown her infant tub and is strong enough to sit up by herself, she is ready for a standard-size bathtub. For babies between six months and twelve months of age, don't run more than a few inches of water into the tub. Be sure to test the water with the inside of your wrist or elbow before lowering baby into the tub. As your child grows, you can adjust the water level accordingly; however, keep it no higher than waist high when your baby is seated in the tub.

To avoid scalds and burns, it is best to keep your baby away from the faucets. Although your baby may not be strong enough to turn on the faucets, little fingers can reach out and touch the water spout. For safety's sake, turn off the hot water first, then continue to run cold water until the spout has cooled off.

SAFETY SMARTS FOR THE TUB

For most children, splashing in the tub is great fun. But as soon as your child is old enough to stand, climb, and reach, the bathtub can pose some serious safety hazards. To prevent slips, falls, scalding, and other bathtub accidents, follow these safety steps.

- Fit your bathtub with a tray to hold bath care items such as soaps, sponges, and shampoo. Or stash them in a plastic bucket on the floor. (Empty the bucket after your child's bath.) The point is to keep toiletries and bathing gear out of reach of little hands.
- If possible, cover the hot and cold water knobs and the spout with inflatable thickly cushioned shields designed to attach to these fixtures. Tub knob and spout covers will protect your child from such bathtub mishaps as bumping her head against the spout, turning on the hot water, and/or touching a hot spout.
- Place a slip-proof rubber mat on the bottom of your tub. Because they cover a large area, mats are safer than adhesive bathtub strips, which leave enough surface unprotected for toddlers to lose their footing and fall.
- Do not allow your little one to stand or kneel in the water. To encourage her to sit, consider a bathtub sitter, a special safety seat designed for babies and toddlers from six months to two years of age. If you opt for a bathtub sitter, you still must never leave your child unattended during her bath.
- Place a slip-proof bath mat on the floor near the tub to catch any drips and splashes of water and to keep your child's feet from sliding on a bare floor. Look for bath mats with thick, absorbent pile and a rubber underbase. A throw rug will not do the trick!
- Fasten safety grip bars to the inside walls of your tub, and teach your child how to hold on to them when getting out of the tub. To help you find safety items for the bathroom,

check *Perfectly Safe,* a free catalog of child safety products. Call 1-800-837-KIDS.

MORE SAFETY SMARTS: TESTING THE WATERS

Concerning bathroom safety, the National Safe Kids Campaign, a child safety organization of the Children's National Medical Center in Washington, D.C., points out that many drownings and near-drownings occur when a child is left alone in the tub. According to the campaign, children under four are at especially high risk.

It takes only an inch of water and a few seconds for a child to drown. In the time it takes to answer the phone or get a towel from the linen closet, your child's life can be in danger. *Never, never, never* leave a small child alone in the tub, not even with an older sibling.

Another bathroom hazard: painful scald burns caused by hot water. While most scald burns happen in the kitchen, the worst ones happen in the bathtub. Hot water (and other hot liquids) burn like fire. In the bathtub, hot water can burn a large area of your child's skin in seconds. And the larger the burn, the more dangerous it is.

As they begin to walk, climb, and reach, toddlers are at the greatest risk of scald burns. No matter how old your children are, it is important to learn how to prevent scalds in the bathroom. Follow these safety tips from the National Safe Kids Campaign:

Test the water temperature of your hot water. Turn on the hot water tap in your tub and let it run for three to five minutes. Using a hot water gauge, a mercury thermometer, or a liquid crystal bath thermometer, measure the temperature of the water. To be safe, hot water should not be hotter than 96 to 100 degrees F.

For safety's sake, check your water heater's thermostat. Set the thermostat to "low," "warm," or 120 degrees F. Wait twenty-four hours, then check the water temperature again. If necessary, repeat this test until the water temperature is safe.

Install antiscald devices in bathtub and shower fixtures. These safety devices use a temperature-sensitive spring to stop the water flow when the temperature goes above 120 degrees F. (*Attention, renters:* Ask your landlord to lower the water temperature of your building's water heater or to fit your bathtub and shower fixtures with antiscald devices.)

Always check the water temperature after filling the tub. Place your entire hand in the water and swish it back and forth for a few seconds. If the water feels even slightly hot, it is too hot for your child's delicate skin. Add more cold water, then repeat the temperature test with the opposite hand. When the bath water feels mildly warm, place your child in the tub.

Again, *always* supervise your kids in the tub. Toddlers can easily turn on the hot water if you don't have tub knob covers. And there's always a chance that an older sibling could accidentally scald a younger child—the buddy system does not apply here. Be on the alert, and bath time can be fun for all!

LITTLE BATHERS AND BUBBLE BATH

A tubful of bubbles is especially inviting to children. However, sometimes bubbles spell trouble. You may have read reports on how bubble bath products may cause urinary tract infections in small children, especially girls.

The ingredient that has been singled out as the potential irritant is the detergent. Although most children's products have been formulated with gentle, nonirritating ingredients, the Food and Drug Administration has proposed labeling all children's bubble bath products with a warning. To date, the labeling issue has not been resolved. Does this mean that you should shelve your child's bubble bath products? Not necessarily. Used with caution, bubbles add fun to the tub.

SAFE BUBBLES

- To play it safe, carefully measure the correct amount of bubble bath to the bath water. (Your child may be overly enthusiastic if allowed to do this on his own!)
- Swish the bubble bath with the bath water to dilute and disperse the product evenly before your child climbs into the tub. (Some dermatologists think it likely that bubble bath poses a problem when the undiluted solu-

tion comes into contact with the skin and mucous membranes.)
- Don't allow a small child to sit in a tub filled with bubbles for more than five minutes or so.
- At the first sign of rash, redness, or itching, discontinue use. If the irritation does not clear up quickly, consult your pediatrician.

BEST BUBBLE BATH BETS

- To protect your child's delicate skin against irritation, choose bubble bath products that are especially formulated for children.
- Read labels. Look for bubble bath that is free of alcohol, which can be drying. Hypoallergenic formulas can help to minimize the risk of allergic reactions.
- Just as you choose a no-tears formula for a baby's or small child's hair, you should choose a bubble bath that won't sting the eyes. Again, check labels.
- Some bubble bath products for kids come in fruity scents such as watermelon or cherry. The eye-pleasing colors and strong fragrances may tempt some children to taste them. Be sure to keep all bubble bath products out of reach and tightly capped when not in use.

SAFETY ALERT!

Unless the label indicates that a bath or shower product is safe for children, please *do not* share your own bath or shower gels, salts, or foaming liquids with your child. Many products made for adults will be labeled "For adult use only" and/or "Keep out of reach of children." Again, keep all bath and shower products out of reach—and out of harm's way.

MAKE YOUR OWN BATH TREATS

For a bath that's gentle on your child's skin, go back to nature and whip up your own bath additives with herbs and essential oils extracted from plants, fruits, and flowers. These natural wonders are used in *aromatherapy*, a down-to-earth beauty and health system that uses fragrant essential oils and herbs to soothe the skin and delight the senses. Try these easy recipes from aromatherapist Judith Jackson, author of *Scentual Touch: A Personal Guide to Aromatherapy*.

The same chamomile tea that relaxes you at bedtime is also a wonderful skin softener when added to your child's bath water. Chamomile has anti-inflammatory properties, making it safe for sensitive skin. Brew a cup of the tea and let it cool to room temperature. Pour half a cup of tea into an infant's bath; use a full cup for an older child. If the tea makes the bath water too warm, run a little cold water until the bath water temperature feels comfortable.

A delightful alternative to bubble bath: Mix one tablespoon of a non-tears formula baby shampoo with three drops of lavender oil. The baby shampoo helps to emulsify the oil, so that it disperses in the water and doesn't just sit on the surface of the skin where it can't do any good. Soothing to the skin, lavender oil has a clean, refreshing scent. Other options include geranium oil and tangerine oil. Essential oils are available at health food stores and specialty bath and apothecary shops such as Caswell-Massey.

To cool your child's sunburn, brew a cup of comfrey tea and stir it into tepid bath water. Comfrey has astringent properties and helps to calm swelling and inflammation.

Note: You may want to check with your pediatrician before trying these recipes if you think that your child may be allergic or sensitive.

SOOTHING SOAKS
TO RELIEVE SKIN CARE WOES

Some of the best bath treatments to soothe dry, flaky, itchy, or inflamed skin can be made with ingredients found in your kitchen or medicine chest. Coming up, a few recipes to help you brew special skin-smoothing baths for your child. (You may even want to try them yourself!)

- For a soothing bath, pour a cup of instant nonfat dry milk powder into a tub of warm water. To disperse the powder, swirl it around until the water turns cloudy. The milk protein softens the water and is gentle on tender skin.
- To relieve a sunburn, toss a cup of white vinegar into a tub of cool water. What helps to pamper dry, flaky skin: a cup of apple cider vinegar poured into a tub of tepid water.
- Another sunburn soother: Fill the tub with tepid water and add a liberal amount of baking soda.
- Colloidal oatmeal, made by dry-milling whole oat kernels into a fine talclike powder, calms a multitude of skin irritations, including diaper rash, prickly heat, eczema, allergic dermatitis, sunburn, insect bites, hives, chicken pox, and measles. It comes in premeasured packets, ready to mix with cool or tepid bath water. This anti-itch treatment is also an excellent cleanser.
- To treat dry skin, add a capful of baby oil to tepid bath water. This is best for children who no longer play with toys in the tub—the oil-laced water can make bath toys sticky! Or you can add the oil during your child's last few minutes in the tub after removing toys.
- Young children may be tempted to sample the water, especially if you add something digestible, such as milk. Whichever additives you choose, watch that your child does not taste or drink the tub water.

More thoughts about soothing your child's skin troubles: Bathing with plain soap can be too harsh on irritated skin. A baby-formula colloidal oatmeal soap or one made for normal-to-dry skin is a gentle alternative.

Another option: Take some colloidal oatmeal and tie it up in a handkerchief or thin sock secured with a rubber band. Next, soak it in cool or tepid water and rub it over your child's skin as you would a sponge or washcloth. Ready-made baby wash bags are available at The

Body Shop, specialty stores carrying natural baby care products. These little sacks are filled with soothing bran, almond meal, oatmeal, and lavender, and meant to be used in lieu of soap and washcloth.

After your child's bath, gently blot her skin with a towel—do not rub—then apply a mild, hypoallergenic body lotion to lock in skin's natural moisture. For skin that is especially itchy or reddened, you may want to try a formula with one percent colloidal oatmeal.

HOW TO GET RELUCTANT KIDS INTO THE TUB

Every now and then you may have to practically arm-wrestle your youngster to get him to take a bath. This resistance to the bathing ritual seems to be part of growing up and testing boundaries. Here are a few ways to make tub time easier on you and more fun for your child.

- Make bath time a rule. Kids are less apt to challenge you if certain activities are set as rules, activities they can expect. Running your child's bath at the same time each day will help.
- Make bath time a ritual. One way to ease your child into the bath is to allow her to choose a few favorite tub toys to keep her company. Give your child a treat to look forward to after her bath. Read her a story or sing a lullaby. Whatever activity you choose, make it clear that it is part of your child's bath time ritual.
- Use a little psychology to "soft-soap" your youngster. Example:

YOU: "Do you want to take a bath?"
CHILD: "No!"
YOU: "Well, would you like to play with some bubbles?"
CHILD: "Yes!"

Instead of insisting on your own way, give your child a choice. Example:

YOU: "The longer it takes for you to get into the tub, the less time we'll have for a story. It's up to you!" Chances are that your child will go for the tub!

- Turn rub-a-dubbing into a game. What makes a splash with kids: Pop-up sponges in whimsical animal shapes. Special story books made to be taken into the tub. For children ages three and up there are colorful fingerpaint gel soaps as well as light and airy foam soaps that whoosh out of a can. And for little doodlers there are erasable scribbling boards that come with kid-safe soap crayons in bright colors.
- Promise your child a bath by candlelight. Place small votive candles on the vanity of your sink or on a windowsill—well out of reach of small children. Turn off the light, and you transform the room into a fairy kingdom or a mysterious secret cave. Your child will be so enchanted by the warm glow of the dancing flames that she will find the bath to be a magical place. (It goes without saying that you must never leave a small child alone in the room with burning candles.)
- Brighten a dark mood with music. Your child may sing a different tune about bath time if you include music as part of the ritual. Special waterproof transistor radios made for bathrooms are available for this purpose.

SHOWER POWER

Up until the age of eight, many children prefer the tub to the shower. The high pressure of the shower may be too powerful for tender skin. Or your child may prefer being waist-high in bubbles and navigating his bath toys.

However, if Mom and Dad take showers, chances are that your youngster may want to do as you do—before the age of eight. Only you can decide when your child is old enough—and responsible enough—to take a shower. When you feel that he is ready, teach him the ropes of shower safety by getting into the shower with him the first few times.

Showers should be speedy—five minutes is all it takes to shampoo hair and scrub the body from nose to toes. Quick showers are also less drying to the skin. To make the shower safe for your child, follow these accident-prevention tips.

1. To prevent scald burns, install an antiscald device in the shower head as recommended by the National Safe Kids Campaign.
2. Fasten safety grip bars to the shower walls. Should your youngster lose her balance while showering, she can grab the bar to prevent falling.
3. Place a nonskid rubber bath mat on the floor of the shower.
4. Stash soaps, shampoo, and other shower necessities in an easy-to-reach shower caddy—never on the floor of the shower. Some shower curtains are designed with self-draining pockets meant to hold bath and shower gear.
5. Your young water bug may have trouble keeping the water in the shower and off the bathroom floor. To keep the spray of water behind the shower curtains, invest in special clip devices designed to hold the curtain taut at the sides and bottom.
6. If you have a glass-enclosed shower stall, make sure that the walls are made of safety glass.

"A LITTLE PRIVACY, PLEASE!"

One day your child is playing in the tub with his floating zoo of bath toys. You're nearby, brushing your teeth or folding towels or just watching him having fun. And then there comes a day when your child turns you out of the bathroom when it's his turn for the tub and bolts the door.

What's going on? Between the ages of seven and ten many children begin to feel a growing need for privacy. They may no longer want you with them in the examination room during a doctor's visit. They may start to hoard "treasures" in secret drawers or keep a diary with a lock and key.

At this age your child has a need to define her separateness, and getting private time in the bathroom is one way of doing so. Your growing child's body begins to go through changes that she may find at turns bewildering and fascinating. Children may want privacy simply to gaze at their reflections in the mirror for more signs of these exciting changes.

The middle years of childhood help to set the stage for adolescence. Time alone in the bathroom gives your child an opportunity to explore her body, play with hairstyles, or to just let her thoughts and imagination wander freely as she lolls in the tub—without the intrusion of an approving or disapproving adult.

This shift in behavior may make you feel left out at times. But your child is not rejecting you, nor is he becoming abnormally preoccupied with his body. He is on a journey of self-discovery, and becoming familiar with the changes in his body is part of that voyage. Your child will feel more secure if you show a healthy respect for his need for privacy. And if you haven't already, you may want to initiate some open discussions with your child about his budding sexuality and what lies ahead.

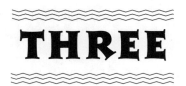

THREE

Bites, Bumps, and Sunburn: Skin Care for the Great Outdoors

P LAYING OUTDOORS IN the fresh air and sunshine of a beautiful day is one of the joys of childhood. But very often these pleasures come to a halt when your child comes home from a camping trip with a case of poison ivy or returns from the beach with a nasty sunburn. This chapter will tell you how to keep your child's skin safe in the great outdoors and how to treat any minor mishaps.

We'll look at smart ways to protect your child's skin against sun damage, including how to choose a gentle sunscreen and how to scope out the best shady hats and sunglasses for kids. This chapter also includes soothing natural remedies to cool a sunburn plus a plan to help you spot changes in your child's skin (and your own) that may lead to skin cancer.

To keep your child covered when your family hits the nature trail there are pointers on poison ivy, including how to avoid it and how to treat this annoying rash. You'll also find tips on how to relieve bee and wasp stings, how to soothe insect and tick bites, what precautions to take against Lyme disease, and how to use insect repellents safely. So, whether your child is hiking, swimming, camping, or just exploring the wilds of your own backyard, you'll be prepared for almost any skin care emergency—and everyone in your family will have more time for outdoor fun!

SUNPROOF YOUR KIDS: HOW TO PROTECT CHILDREN AGAINST SUN DAMAGE

Did you know that one blistering sunburn during childhood may more than double the risk of developing melanoma (the deadliest form of skin cancer) later in life?

You may be surprised to learn that both freckles and the golden glow of a tan that look so healthy are signs of sun damage. Sunlight triggers the formation of melanin, which forms a tan and/or freckles. While a tan is the skin's natural defense against further damage, melanin forms as a result of the skin's being *injured* by the sun. Your skin's natural repair mechanisms go into action to heal such injuries, but there is no medical evidence that they can undo all the damage.

Over the years chronic exposure to sunlight leads to wrinkling, discoloring, and premature aging of the skin. Even black and other dark skin tones, which are less susceptible to burning, are vulnerable to these harmful effects of the sun, including skin cancer.

As a parent you should be aware that sun damage is cumulative and builds up with each reexposure. The skin has a long memory and does not forget an insult! Unless you take steps now to protect your child's skin, eventually the natural repair system breaks down. If unprotected skin is repeatedly injured, abnormal cells build up; when these cells accumulate at an uncontrollable rate, skin cancer is the result.

Does this mean that you have to keep your child locked up indoors? Not at all. Your child can still have fun in the sun if you play it safe. Begin now and you can beat the odds against the most common skin cancers by 78 percent. Herewith, some good sun sense for children.

GOLDEN RULES OF SUN PROTECTION

- Keep infants out of direct sunlight. It's an excellent idea to fit your baby's or toddler's stroller with a protective canopy or

umbrella. A carriage with a hood helps to keep infants out of harm's way.
- Do not use sunscreen on infants under six months of age without consulting your physician. A baby's skin is quite transparent and penetrable; it is not known how the penetration of strong sunscreen chemicals can affect a baby's body system. According to medical experts, it takes about six months for an infant's skin to develop enough so that it can tolerate a sunscreen.
- In lieu of using sunscreen, dress your infant in protective clothing including a broad-brimmed hat. Tightly woven fabrics that breathe, such as cotton, are best. Be sure to cover arms and legs. And opt for double layers when possible.
- Take precautions against reflected light. Sand reflects up to 25 percent of harmful ultraviolet rays, snow up to 85 percent, and water up to 85 percent. The ultraviolet rays that bounce off these surfaces add to the radiation that you get from direct sunlight. On a cloudy or overcast day you still get as much as 80 percent of the sun's radiation. Sun protection is a must!
- It's a good idea to place your baby's carriage or stroller on the grass (in the shade, of course!) rather than on a patio, which is a more reflective surface. For trips to the beach, don't sit close to the water; place the stroller or carriage on your beach blanket rather than on the sand.
- For children older than six months, *do* apply a sunscreen every time your child spends time outdoors. The Skin Cancer Foundation and the American Academy of Dermatology recommend a sunscreen with an SPF (Sun Protection Factor) of 15. This means that your child's skin is protected against sun damage fifteen times longer than it would be without a sunscreen. A sunscreen with an SPF of 15 filters out 93 to 94 percent of the sun's UVB (ultraviolet B) rays, the so-called "burning" rays. Check labels to make sure it also filters out the longer UVA (ultraviolet A) rays, the so-called "tanning" rays.
- The safest sunning hours are during the early morning or late afternoon. The sun's rays are most intense between 10 A.M. and 2 P.M. (11 A.M. to 3 P.M. Daylight Savings Time).

- While all children, including those with dark hair and deep skin tones, are at risk for sun damage, your child is especially vulnerable if he or she has fair skin that freckles or burns easily, blond or red hair, and light eyes. Try to plan outdoor gym activities, tennis lessons, or visits to the park during the morning or late afternoon.
- When you send your child off to daycare, nursery school, kindergarten, or camp, pack a sunscreen with his or her belongings. Inform the teacher or instructor and ask that the sunscreen be applied before any outdoor activities.
- If you live at high altitudes or in the Sunbelt, you need to be especially careful about sun protection. For every 1,000 feet above sea level, ultraviolet radiation increases by 4 to 5 percent. And the closer you are to the equator, the more intense the sun's rays are.

For more information on sun protection for children send for the free brochure, "Sunproofing Your Baby." Write to The Skin Cancer Foundation, P.O. Box 561, New York, NY 10156.

SUN STUFF: SUNSCREENS FOR CHILDREN

When buying sunscreen for your child, check labels. Look for alcohol-free formulas. (Alcohol can irritate young skin.) Sunscreens for children should also be fragrance free (fragrance can attract insects as well as irritate tender skin) and allergy-tested. (The label may also say "dermatologist-tested," which means that a skin doctor has tested the sunscreen to determine whether or not the product *generally* causes allergic reactions.)

Many sunscreens for children use the word *baby* on the label. However, if you take the time to read the fine print on the label you will see that they are not meant to be used on babies under six months of age.

Although only 7 percent of the population is allergic to PABA, a common sunscreen agent, you may want to choose PABA-free formulas for your child. If you prefer PABA-free sunscreens, avoid those with Padimate A and Padimate O, derivatives of PABA. Check labels!

When shopping for sunscreens, you may notice that some products carry the seal of recommendation from The Skin Cancer Foundation. This seal is given to those sunscreens with an SPF of 15 or greater that meet the stringent criteria set by the foundation's Photobiology Committee. The following guide will help you to choose a gentle sunscreen for your child.

Whether your child is splashing in the backyard pool or running through the sprinkler, consider a waterproof formula. Waterproof sunscreens bond to the skin so that your child won't swim off (or sweat off) the sunscreen. *Waterproof* protection lasts for eighty minutes in the water. *Water-resistant* sunscreens hold up for forty minutes.

If you have a wriggly kid who won't sit still long enough for you to apply sunscreen, spritz on one of the new spray-on formulas. (Kids seem to find spray-ons more fun, too.) Make sure the product is alcohol free, though. And be careful not to get any spray into eyes.

For active kids, new sports formulas are light, nonsticky, and absorb quickly without leaving any residue. One great advantage: there's less chance the sunscreen will run into your children's eyes when they perspire.

Another choice for on-the-go kids: sunscreen towelettes. These handy foil-wrapped towelettes are soaked with a PABA-free sunscreen. Compact and portable, towelettes are great to stash in your beach bag or to take along on picnics and family outings.

The nose, cheeks, ears, and scalp where the hair is parted are especially sun-sensitive. Sunscreen in neat stick form is excellent for on-the-spot protection. For burn-prone cheeks and the nose, zinc oxide provides an opaque physical sunblock. And now zinc oxide comes in neon-bright colors kids love! Don't worry—it comes off with soap and water.

There is now sunscreen for children made with *titanium dioxide*, an invisible barrier that blocks out burning ultraviolet-B rays and damaging ultraviolet-A rays. Most sunscreen ingredients are chemical. Titanium dioxide works by reflecting or scattering ultraviolet rays and is said to be gentler on sensitive skin than chemical sunscreens.

Another gentle formula: no-tears sunscreens. Wonderful for small children, they won't sting sensitive eyes.

Slick your child's lips with a lip balm containing sunscreen. This is important because lips have no protective melanin and burn fastest if not shielded against the sun. Lip sunscreens for kids also come in yummy flavors.

For youngsters ages six and up, there are water-resistant stick sunscreens that leave a sparkly sheen on the body. If you do opt for this formula, be sure that the one you choose has an SPF of 15 or higher—some shimmery sunscreens don't. *Note:* The light-reflecting sparkles in the formula are inert particles and therefore should not irritate young skin.

PATCH-TESTING HOW-TOS FOR SUNSCREEN

As you already know, sensitivity to any skin care product is highly individual. Whatever sunscreen formula you choose, it is a good idea to patch-test the product before use. Darrell S. Rigel, M.D., Clinical Associate Professor of Dermatology at New York University, suggests the following procedure for patch-testing:

1. Apply a small amount of sunscreen to an area of skin about the size of a nickel on the inside of your child's arm. To keep the sunscreen from rubbing off, cover the area with a nonstick adhesive bandage.
2. After ten to twenty minutes, check the skin. An *immediate* positive reaction will be characterized by redness, blotchiness, or a fine, red bumpy rash accompanied by a stinging pins-and-needles sensation.
3. If there is no immediate reaction, cover the area and check it again after twenty-four to forty-eight hours. A *delayed* reaction may occur. This is characterized by a red, itchy rash with large bumps (each bump being approximately $\frac{1}{8}$ of an inch in size).
4. Whether your child experiences an immediate reaction or delayed reaction, discard the product. You may want to consult your pediatrician for advice on other products.

SUNSCREEN APPLICATION HOW-TOS

Your child's sunscreen will give the best results if you follow these easy instructions.

When you find a sunscreen that your child can tolerate, apply it liberally. Do not skimp! Smooth it over all exposed skin, being careful not to get it too close to the eyes. It is also a good idea to apply sunscreen under sheer or thin clothing, including wet T-shirts.

To give sunscreen ingredients a chance to go to work, apply sunscreen fifteen to thirty minutes before your child heads outdoors. And be careful to reapply it often throughout the day. For a sunscreen to be effective, it must be applied to dry (not wet or damp) skin. Once your child is out of the water (or has been perspiring), reapply sunscreen after towel-drying skin.

If your child is taking medication, check with your doctor before letting him go out in the sun. Some antibiotics such as tetracycline and erythromycin don't mix well with sunlight. One side effect may be *photosensitivity*—an adverse reaction to sun exposure characterized by rash, redness, and/or swelling.

NATURAL SOOTHERS FOR SUNBURN

As discussed in chapter 1, a baby's skin is especially vulnerable to sunburn (see "TLC for Newborn Skin," pages 7–8). If your baby is under one year old and gets a sunburn, call your doctor immediately. You also need to call the doctor for a child one year old or older if she seems to have intense pain, has a fever over 101 degrees F, seems lethargic, or has a second-degree burn (blisters on the outer layer of skin).

What can you do until you can see the doctor? Or, how do you treat less severe sunburns that don't require professional medical care? Relief is on the way if you try these soothing treatments:

- Three to four times a day apply wet compresses of cool tap water. Cool compresses ease the pain and reduce redness and swelling.

- Skin care pro Lia Schorr of Lia Schorr Skin Care Salon in New York City suggests applying compresses of cold milk to sunburned areas. Dip cotton into milk and place on skin for twenty minutes; reapply as needed. Or, if it's practical, slather on plain yogurt. The yogurt helps to calm the burning sensation as it refreshes the skin. After twenty minutes rinse off with cool water and pat dry.
- Take the leaf of an aloe plant, snip the tip, and squeeze the natural aloe gel into the palm of your hand. Smooth it over sunburned area. The aloe helps to reduce redness as it heals the burn.
- To soothe and refresh small areas of sunburned skin, apply thin slices of raw cucumber, potato, or apple.
- Another practical sunburn-soother for small areas: cornstarch. Mix cornstarch with enough water to make a paste; apply the mixture. Remove with cool water after twenty minutes.
- To soften taut, dry skin and promote healing, apply a lubricating lotion or cream. Caution: medicated creams, including those containing hydrocortisone and benzocaine, should not be used on babies without consulting your pediatrician first. Do not use greasy, occlusive emollients, which clog pores and trap heat.
- Use a light touch to massage in creams or lotions. If this seems to be too painful for your child, skip applying creams or lotions until your child's skin is less tender.
- Give your child acetaminophen as recommended by your doctor if your child's temperature is above 101 degrees F or to relieve sunburn pain.
- Have your child drink plenty of water to replace lost body fluids.
- Wait until your child's skin has healed before letting him or her go out in the sun. Contrary to popular belief, once skin has been burned, it is more vulnerable to a second sunburn.
- Once your child is ready to resume playing outdoors, be diligent about applying sunscreen and taking other sun safety precautions. Cumulative damage caused by repeated overexposure to sunlight cannot be reversed.

SAFETY CHECK FOR SKIN

Although skin cancer is rare in children and uncommon in teenagers, it pays to be on the lookout for any early warning signs. Doing a routine check of your child's skin will teach concern for skin care at an early age and encourage your child to do the same later in life, a habit that can be truly life saving! (Early detection and treatment can cure skin cancer.) Though a child who is fair and/or has a lot of moles is at highest risk, children of all coloring should be checked. Regular examination is recommended by The Skin Cancer Foundation and the American Academy of Dermatology as follows:

- When you bathe your child, carefully examine his or her skin for any changes. What to watch for: New raised growths; itchy patches; nonhealing sores; changes in moles; or new colored areas. Any of these changes should be discussed with your doctor.
- When inspecting moles watch for any changes in their sizes, shapes, edges, and color. Think A-B-C-D—for *Asymmetry, Border, Color,* and *Diameter*. The following guide based on the warning signs developed by the American Academy of Dermatology will help you to tell the difference between normal, benign moles and early malignant melanoma.

THE ABCD'S OF BENIGN MOLES

Asymmetry: Moles are round and symmetrical.
Border: Moles have even edges.
Color: One shade of brown.
Diameter: Smaller than 6 mm.

THE ABCD'S OF MALIGNANT MELANOMA

Asymmetry: One half of the mole does not match the other half.

Border: Edges are uneven, scalloped, or notched.
Color: Two or more shades of tan, brown, or black.
Diameter: Larger than 6 mm (the size of a pencil eraser).

Again, while the odds of getting skin cancer during childhood are low, being on the alert gives your children a head start in keeping their skin healthy for a lifetime.

WE'VE GOT YOU COVERED: HINTS ON HATS

For babies and older children alike, a tightly woven hat with a broad brim helps to keep sunlight off the face. When choosing a hat for your child, follow these tips.

- Avoid straw hats. Designed with an openwork wicker weave, they are likely to let in more sunlight than a closely woven fabric hat.
- Baseball caps are "in" now, but this hot item does little to sunproof the face and ears. Your child needs a hat with a protective all-around brim.
- To shade your child's head, face, ears, and neck, a hat brim should be at least three inches wide and extend around all sides—not just the front.

CHOOSING SUNGLASSES FOR CHILDREN

Just as sunlight can damage your children's skin, too much sun can take its toll on their eyes. Eye researchers believe that age-related retinal disease, a cause of blindness affecting 24 percent of adults over the age of sixty, may have its origins in exposure to sunlight during childhood. According to eye-care expert Jack Weber, O.D., director of education and research at Marchon & Marcolin Eyewear, "It is in childhood, when the eyes' lenses are clear, that solar radiation can reach the retina far more easily than it does during adulthood."

To protect your children's eyes, Dr. Weber recommends that they wear a large-brimmed hat or visor to shade the eyes and face *and* a pair of protective sunglasses. Wearing good-quality sunglasses also protects sensitive eyelids against burning and keeps your child from squinting.

Unfortunately, more than 50 percent of the children's sunglasses available over the counter today do not provide adequate protection against ultraviolet light. To pick a pair of sun-safe sunglasses, follow these simple steps:

Invest in lenses made of unbreakable polycarbonate. Check the label to make sure that the lenses provide protection against both UVB (ultraviolet B) and UVA (ultraviolet A) rays. *Note:* The Food and Drug Administration (FDA) has approved a voluntary labeling system (for nonprescription sunglass lenses) developed by the Sunglass Association of America. The label tells you how much UV protection you're getting from the lenses.

Choose the highest level of protection for your child. The label might read, "Exceeds ANSI [American National Standards Institute] Z-80.3 UV requirements for sunglasses maximum UV protection." These lenses filter out at least 99 percent of UVB rays, at least 60 percent of UVA rays, and 20 to 97 percent of visible light.

If you prefer not to go label hunting in the drugstore, you can go to your optometrist's office or a good optical shop and have the lenses of your child's sunglasses treated with a coating that absorbs 99 percent of UVB and 99 percent of UVA rays.

For eye comfort, consider color. *Gray* lenses, which do not distort the colors red and blue, offer the best color perception. *Green* lenses have some minor color distortion but are easy on the eyes. And *amber* and *brown* lenses are better at filtering out ultraviolet light.

Avoid blue lenses. Blue light rays, which scatter through the atmosphere, cause "visual static," causing objects to look flat and fuzzy. Blue lenses make this static worse.

If your child has dark eyes, lenses in medium-to-light colors will feel the most comfortable. (Dark eyes have more pigment than lighter eyes, which helps to absorb brightness.) Light eyes are more light-sensitive. Children with light eyes will feel better wearing darker lenses. Whether your child's eyes are light or dark, they need sunglasses with UV inhibitors.

To check lenses for flaws, look for waves and bubbles. Standing by a window, hold the sunglasses a few inches away from your eyes. Make sure the window frame does not distort your view.

POINTERS ON POISON IVY

The itching and burning of poison ivy may be one of your all-too-familiar childhood memories. To minimize the misery of poison ivy for your child it helps to know exactly what causes this rash.

Poison ivy, poison oak, and poison sumac are part of the *rhus* (poison ivy) plant family. When cut or crushed, all parts of the rhus plant exude an oily resin called *urushiol*, which contains powerful allergens. Coming into contact with this oil exposes skin to the allergens that trigger the poison ivy rash.

If your child is sensitive to the poison ivy allergens she may get a reaction within twelve to forty-eight hours of exposure. The symptoms: redness and swelling, then blisters and intense itching. After a few days the blisters form crusts and begin to scale. Poison ivy takes about ten days to heal—an eternity for both parent and child—and can leave small pigmented spots, particularly if your child's skin is dark.

The severity and extent of your child's reaction depends on three things:

1. How allergic he is.
2. How much of the poison ivy oil (resin) has been deposited on his skin.
3. How much of the skin has been exposed to the poison ivy oil (resin).

Be aware that poison ivy can occur on almost any part of the body. Areas where the skin is thinner, such as the backs of hands, tend to be more vulnerable, whereas the palms of hands and soles of feet are less prone to react with a rash.

Treating Poison Ivy

If you know that your child has been in contact with poison ivy, poison oak, or poison sumac, wash away the sap as soon as possible with cold running water. Use a garden hose if one is handy. If you're having a picnic or camping, it may be convenient to douse your child in a nearby stream or lake. The point is to act quickly. Rinsing the skin within five minutes of exposure will neutralize the resin in the plant's sap and keep it from spreading. However, if you can't react this swiftly, don't panic. Chances are that if you can wash away the resin within thirty minutes of exposure, you can at least lessen the intensity of any poison ivy flare-up, if not stop the development of a reaction altogether.

Be sure to rinse your child's hands. Be thorough and cleanse the skin under the fingernails. Any traces of resin under the nails can be spread to other parts of the body.

You should also launder your child's clothing, since it most likely came into contact with the poison ivy plant. Try to wash clothing outdoors with a garden hose before you bring it into your house so that you don't track resin onto your furniture or carpeting.

If your child's skin does break out in a poison ivy rash, follow these simple steps:

- Apply cool water compresses where needed to relieve itching and calm redness. Cool baths are also soothing.
- To speed up the drying of small blisters apply calamine lotion. Give your child a tepid bath with colloidal oatmeal to soothe and help heal blisters as well as reduce itchiness.
- Try to discourage your child from scratching blisters. Germs often find snug hiding places under fingernails, and the germs can infect the broken blisters. If an infection does occur, your pediatric dermatologist can prescribe antibiotics for your child.
- If your child's case of poison ivy seems severe, consult a pediatric dermatologist. An intense bout of poison ivy can be treated with local or systemic corticosteroids.

Preventing Poison Ivy

"Leaves of three—let them be." During your childhood you may have learned this rhyme and used it as your guide in avoiding poison ivy. However, there are many exceptions to this rule. The leaflets of poison ivy and poison oak may grow in groups of three, or groups of five, seven, or nine.

HERE'S LOOKING AT YOU, KID!

Since the best way to prevent poison ivy is to avoid contact with the plants, learn to know what they look like. And teach your child to be on the lookout for these plants as soon as she is old enough to learn.

To help you recognize poison ivy, poison oak, and poison oak, follow these guidelines from the American Academy of Dermatology.

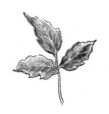

Poison Ivy: The plant has yellow-green flowers and white berries. Leaflets grow in groups of three or groups of five, seven, and nine. It grows east of the Rocky Mountains. It also grows as a low shrub near the Great Lakes and in the northern states; as a vine or climbing vine in the East, Midwest, and South.

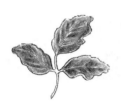

Poison Oak: The plant has clusters of yellow berries. Leaflets that resemble oak tree leaves grow in groups of three or groups of five, seven, or nine. It grows as a shrub in the East; as a vine and low shrub in the West and Southwest.

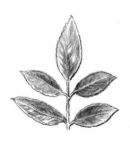

Poison Sumac: The plant grows as a tall, spindly shrub with cream-colored berries. Each leaf bears seven to thirteen leaflets with smooth edges. It crops up in standing water in peat bogs in northern states east of the Mississippi River and in swampy areas of parts of the Southeast.

(Illustrations adapted courtesy of the American Academy of Dermatology.)

If you do plan a family outing in an area where you suspect poison ivy plants grow, dress your child in long pants and tops with long sleeves. And don't let your pet romp through the woods. Remember, the poison ivy resin can stick to almost any surface, including the fur of animals.

Bites, Bumps, and Sunburn

RELIEF FOR BEE AND WASP STINGS

Ouch! As soon as your child is stung by a bee or wasp, she feels pain and a burning sensation. Swelling and itching follow. Be aware that a wasp removes its stinger from the skin, but a bee can leave its stinger and venom sac behind. To the rescue, the following tips:

- If the bee sinks its stinger and venom sac in your child's skin, you must remove them. Do not squeeze the skin! Putting pressure on the sac will release more bee venom.
- Do use a pair of tweezers with sharp, pointed prongs, or simply use your fingernails to pull out the stinger and sac.
- To soothe the itching and decrease swelling, apply calamine lotion to the bite site. A simple paste of baking soda and warm water also offers relief. Another simple skin-soother: a cool compress or ice bag applied for ten minutes.
- If your child can tolerate oral antihistamines they may help to stop the itching of the sting.

If Your Child Is Allergic

For most children, bee and wasp stings do not pose a serious threat. However, in some cases, a child can have a severe allergic reaction. Symptoms include:

- Abnormal swelling
- Massive hives
- Wheezing or difficulty in breathing
- Irregular heartbeat
- Diarrhea
- Shock (drop in blood pressure; cold, clammy skin; fast, weak pulse; dilated pupils)

If your child shows signs of a severe reaction, a doctor's immediate attention is a must! Take your child to the emergency room if necessary. Allergy shots to desensitize your child may be in order.

Be prepared for emergencies. When you pack for a picnic or any outdoor activity, take along a bee or wasp sting kit (called an *anaphylaxis kit*). This precaution is especially important if your child is allergic to insect bites. The kit should include an antihistamine to counteract itching and shots of *epinephrine* as prescribed by your doctor to reduce swelling. Injecting this potent medication constricts blood vessels. Keep a kit at home and in your car.

DOS AND DON'TS FOR PREVENTING BEE STINGS

Your child will be less of a target for bees if you take the following steps:

Do dress your child in white or light-colored clothing if you suspect bees are nearby. (A bee's habitat includes flowers, shrubs, beaches, and picnic areas.) Bees seem to be attracted to dark colors.

Don't apply scented skin care products such as body lotions or fragranced sunscreen to your child's skin. The aroma seems to be irresistible to bees. Opt for fragrance-free skin care products and hair care products.

Don't allow your child to go barefoot outdoors if bees are buzzing nearby. This may not always be practical (for example, at the beach), but following this step will minimize the risk of getting stung by any bees underfoot—a common scenario.

WHAT TO DO ABOUT INSECT AND TICK BITES

Mosquitoes, chiggers, ticks: these tiny pests are part of outdoor living, especially in the woods or hot, humid areas. Here's what to do if the bugs bite.

Coping with Chigger Bites

The American red bugs called chiggers are harvest mites and are found throughout the United States. Unlike ticks, chiggers do not burrow into the skin and will fall off the skin without any special treatment. Chigger bites, however, cause extreme discomfort. Symptoms include itching, redness, hives, and possibly blisters.

If your child is bitten by chiggers, put her into a bath as soon as possible to help wash them off the skin. To relieve itching and redness try a cool compress or apply calamine lotion. In severe cases your child may need medication such as antihistamines and topical and/or oral steroids as prescribed by your doctor. To treat an extreme reaction see your pediatrician promptly!

Soothing Mosquito and Fly Bites

As harmless as a mosquito or fly bite is, it can be a nuisance. A small child may be tempted to scratch the red, itchy bumps, so you'll want to take the itch out of the bite. For relief, reach for cool compresses and calamine lotion. If the bite is near the eyes or genitals, skip the calamine lotion, which could spread to and irritate these sensitive areas.

Like bees, mosquitoes are attracted to sweet scents such as those found in perfumed soaps and shampoos. Again, opt for fragrance-free skin care and hair care products. And avoid dressing your child in bright colors, which are very attractive to mosquitoes.

Taking Care of Tick Bites

Tiny ticks can cause big trouble. By now you know that ticks, usually carried by deer and mice, can transmit Lyme disease, a bacterial infection that can lead to arthritis, paralysis, and heart disease. (The number of ticks that carry other infections is also on the rise in the United States.) These troublemakers make their home in wooded and grassy areas as well as shrubs, vines, and bushes.

Your child is probably more at risk than you are simply because he is outdoors more often. However, anyone in your family, including your pets, can contract Lyme disease. Ticks can hide in your child's hair or burrow into the skin. Because they are so tiny, they are difficult to detect. It is important to do a head-to-toe inspection of your child's skin and hair. Be sure to do a thorough check of your child's scalp and nape of the neck.

If you discover that your child has been bitten by a tick, remove it as soon as possible. Removing the tick within twenty-four hours of the bite minimizes the risk of getting Lyme disease. Using a pair of sharp, pointed tweezers, grasp the tick's body near the head and pull it all the way out. Suppose the head breaks off? Get medical help as quickly as you can. To prevent the onset of infection, you need to remove both the head and body.

Next, carefully wash the bite site as well as your hands and your child's hands. A cool compress or calamine lotion will soothe any soreness. Have your child checked by your pediatrician and, if possible, bring the offending tick.

Signs of Lyme Disease

To be on the safe side, check your child for symptoms of Lyme disease. According to the American Academy of Dermatology, the first symptom is a circular red rash that appears around the tick bite within thirty days of infection. This rash flares up in 70 percent of Lyme disease cases. Other symptoms resembling the flu (fatigue, fever, sore throat, aching joints and muscles) can show up within a few days to a few weeks after the tick bite. If detected and treated early enough, Lyme disease will not cause permanent damage. The treatment: antibiotics taken for about ten days.

Preventing Tick Bites

Dressing your child in light-colored clothing makes it easier to spot ticks. Your child should also wear long pants tucked snugly into socks. Applying an insect repellent to your child's clothing and exposed skin also helps to ward off ticks. You want to be certain that your insect repellent is safe, however, so be sure to get your pediatrician's approval.

INSECT REPELLENTS: USE WITH CAUTION

Insect repellent does offer protection against ticks, chiggers, and pesky insects such as mosquitoes and flies. In general, insect repellents with the ingredient *deet* (diethyltoluamide) are recommended. However, experts agree that repellents should not be used on small children unless they will be in areas where insect activity is intense. Infants in particular are vulnerable to allergic reactions. If you do opt for using an insect repellent, choose one with the lowest effective concentration of deet, and be sure to get your pediatrician's approval.

Never spritz the repellent directly on your child's skin. For safe, neat application, spray the repellent into the palm of your hand and then stroke it over your child's skin. Avoid areas near the eyes and mouth.

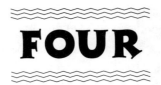

FOUR

Hair Today: Tips for Shining Hair and a Healthy Scalp

WHO IS NOT charmed by the natural beauty of a child's hair as it catches the golden rays of the sun? Whether ruffled by a breeze or tousled by play, silky, healthy, shining hair is key to your child's good looks—and does wonders for his self-esteem. You know what a boost it is to your own confidence when your hair looks great? It's the same with children. Luckily, it is easy to keep your child's hair in beautiful condition, and this chapter will guide you through the basics.

Most of us have learned our hair care habits from our parents. I can still conjure up the fresh, clean fragrance of the shampoo my mother used, and how good it felt to have her fingertips massage my scalp as she gently worked the lather through my hair. But sometimes our lessons were less than pleasant. Do you remember getting shampoo suds in your eyes? The tearful tug of war you went through when Mom or Dad had to comb the knots out of your damp and tangled hair? Or when they had to struggle with the wad of chewing gum stuck in your tresses? Fortunately, there are ways to avoid these ordeals, and we'll go through them in this chapter. By the end you'll be able to glide through the routines of hair care without a snag.

Along with simple steps for shampooing without tears, snarl-free combing, and child-safe conditioning tips for healthy hair, you will also find solutions to common hair care woes such as taming flyaway hair, smoothing the frizzies, and washing away chlorine. And there's help for coping with more troubling hair and scalp problems such as head lice, ringworm, and hair loss. Now it's your turn to pass on your hair care know-how to your child.

HOW HAIR CHANGES

The color and texture of your child's hair is not necessarily fixed at birth. Some babies are born with a thick head of long, silky hair. Others have the barest bit of pale peach fuzz. And some babies born with straight hair grow up to have a tumble of curls.

Perhaps your baby has lost her first crop of head hair during infancy. This sudden hair loss is due to a shift from the *anagen*, or growing, stage of the hair's growth cycle to the *telogen*, or resting, stage when hairs are shed. As unsettling as this may be, it is nothing to worry about. The hair usually grows back within six months to a year. However, it may be a different color or texture because of changes in the makeup of your baby's hair.

The texture and curl pattern of your child's hair during childhood are usually set by the age of three or four. At this time you will see whether or not your child's hair will be straight or curly, fine or coarse—or in between. When the hormones of puberty kick in (around the age of twelve for most children), the texture and curl pattern can go through more changes. As your child grows up, hair color can also fade or darken. This happens when the production of pigments that result in light colors such as blond or red shut down and the production of darker shades steps up.

THE BASICS FOR HEALTHY HAIR

A minilesson in the anatomy of a strand of hair will help you to learn the basics of hair care. While the root of the hair is living, each strand of hair is composed of dead, hardened cells filled with a protein called *keratin*. This protein is the same substance that makes up the epidermis, the outermost layer of the skin. During each growth cycle, the hair shaft is pushed up the follicle toward the scalp at a rate of one-third to one-half inch a month.

Each strand of hair is composed of three layers. The innermost layer is called the *medulla*. Its function is unknown. In fact, the medulla is sometimes missing in otherwise perfectly healthy hair. The middle layer, which contains the granules of pigment that color the hair, is called the *cortex*. Physical changes in the cortex give hair its natural wave. The cortex also retains the water hair needs to stay soft and supple. This essential layer determines the hair's strength and elasticity, the diameter of the hair shaft, and the texture. How hair behaves depends on the structure of the cortex.

The outermost layer is the *cuticle*. A look under a powerful electron microscope would show you that the overlapping cells that form the cuticle resemble shingles on a roof. The cuticle works as a barrier against the everyday wear and tear of combing, brushing, blow-drying, and styling as well as any chemicals that could damage the core of the hair. This layer also helps to seal in the hair's water supply. Without enough water, hair becomes dull and brittle and has no bounce.

What Makes Hair Shiny and Soft

When the clear, shinglelike cells of the cuticle lie flat and intact along the hair shaft, the light that hits this smooth surface bounces off. (Think of how a calm pool of water reflects sunlight.) Hair also feels silky when the cells of the cuticle are smooth and tight, and is less apt to tangle.

Oil glands that open into each follicle produce *sebum*. This natural oil travels up the follicle to lightly coat each strand of hair. This coating of oil works like a natural conditioner to keep water in the hair shaft from evaporating too quickly. And as oil fills in the cracks in the cuticle, it smooths out the surface of the hair shaft.

Healthy, straight hair tends to be shinier than curlier hair. That's because straight hair lies closer to the head, allowing it to be coated more evenly by the scalp's natural oils. Curly hair, which stands up from the scalp, gets less lubrication from the scalp's natural oils.

Curly or Straight, All Hair Types Are Great!

As your child grows up, one hair type or the other may be all the rage at school or among his or her peers. If your child's hair doesn't fit in with the in crowd, he or she may feel inferior. It is important to help your child develop a healthy sense of self-esteem. Compliment your child. Help your youngster to appreciate the unique quality of his or her hair.

When I was in grade school, the long, stick-straight hair of the golden California surfer girl was the up-to-the-minute look. My own hair was—and is—naturally curly, and I felt hopelessly out of it. I was constantly teased by my schoolmates, who called me glamorous names such as "Mop Top."

My parents did their best to soothe my bruised ego. Since my hair had a mind of its own, my dad began to call me "The girl with the magic hair." At first I openly resisted this attempt to mend the chips in my self-esteem. But in a funny way, my dad's playful gesture always made me feel better. Like a small jewel, this memory is tucked away in the treasure chest of my past.

If your child tends to shrug off compliments, focus on what she *does* like about her hair. Ask, "Do you like the color?" "Do you like the way your hair shines when it's just shampooed?" "Do you like the way it feels when you toss your head?" A generous dose of reassurance from Mom and Dad can go a long way in boosting your child's confidence. Straight, curly, or in between, each hair type has it special beauty and with proper care can be your child's crowning glory.

What Damages Hair

Any process or treatment that roughs up the cuticle of the hair shaft causes damage. Everyday brushing, combing, and blow-drying puts stress on your child's hair. Overexposure to sunlight also takes its toll. So does swimming in a chlorinated pool or salt water. All can cause the smooth, tight "shingles" to separate; with enough trauma, these cells can also tear.

When the surface of the cuticle is rough and broken, it loses its shine. The uneven surface can no longer reflect light evenly. It also knots and tangles more easily. Split ends are another sign of abuse. Because the shaft of the hair has been weakened, the ends fray and the layers of cells separate.

A child's hair is more fragile than an adult's, and more vulnerable to damage. If it is fine textured, it also snarls and tangles more easily. Think of your child's hair as a delicate fabric such as silk. Like an exquisite piece of silk, your child's hair needs to be washed and dried gently and handled with a light touch. Treating your child's hair with tender loving care will teach him or her to do the same.

SHAMPOO SMARTS

Clean hair is beautiful hair. Perhaps you've started off your child's hair care regime with a no-tears baby shampoo. If you're happy with the results, you may want to continue to use a nonstinging baby formula as your child grows up. You may also want to explore other options. The following tips will guide your choices.

If you prefer a no-tears baby formula, consider one with added conditioning ingredients. While basic baby shampoos are excellent cleansers and won't sting the eyes, they can be drying and cause flyaway hair. Conditioning ingredients soften the hair so that the strands won't lift up and repel each other. Conditioners also make hair easier to comb. For children ages three to ten, try Pert Plus for Kids, a no-tears shampoo with built-in conditioners.

Another choice in the no-tears category is shampoo in a creamy mousse formula. Like whipped cream, the mousse stays put without running, so there's less chance of its dripping into your child's eyes when you wash his hair. Mousse formulas are available for babies and toddlers as well as older kids.

Shampoo for children should be as gentle on the skin as it is on the hair. A mild and moisturizing shampoo such as Paul Mitchell's Baby Don't Cry Shampoo can double as a body cleanser or bubble bath. One ingredient that makes a shampoo kind to skin and hair is *alphabisabolol*, the healing agent found in chamomile. Herbal ingredients such as echinacea, ginseng extract, and lemongrass are soothing.

If your child has sensitive skin, you may want to try a hypoallergenic children's shampoo. Many shampoos list fragrance among the very last ingredients, adding just enough to make the product pleasant to use without irritating skin.

BABY SHAMPOO SUBSTITUTE

Tip: If you've run out of your baby's or children's formula shampoo, try this trick from London-based trichologist Philip Kingsley, author of *The Complete Healthy Hair Book*. Dilute your own shampoo, mixing one part shampoo with three to five parts distilled water (available at your pharmacy). Of course, the shampoo you use must be mild. If your everyday shampoo is for oily hair or dandruff, it will be too harsh for your child's tresses. A moisturizing shampoo or a "light" formula made for fine or frequently washed hair is a better choice. Diluting the shampoo before applying it to your child's hair and scalp will maximize its mildness.

HAIR WASHING WITHOUT TEARS

While some kids love to have you work foamy peaks of lather through their hair, others squirm, shriek, and wriggle in protest, turning shampoo time into a minor skirmish. My friend Kathleen has one solution to quiet her three-year-old son Devon's screams during his shampoo sessions: "Let Daddy take over. Since Daddy doesn't cry, my son finds it easier to cooperate." This section will map out a few more home-tested strategies to take the tears and trauma out of shampooing your child's hair.

Easy how-tos for washing your infant's hair and scalp are described in chapter 2. As you will recall, emphasis is placed on keeping the lather and water out of baby's eyes. Even if you use a no-tears formula, you want to take care that the foam doesn't drip into baby's eyes.

Because baby shampoo doesn't sting, tears don't form to wash away the product. There is still a chance that any product that gets into the eyes and is not rinsed away may cause some irritation. By tilting your baby's head back you can keep shampoo and water away from baby's face and eyes.

Tip for shampoo-shy tots: As soon as your baby is strong enough to sit up by herself, it may not be so easy to keep her head tilted back. Even though a no-tears shampoo won't sting your child's eyes, many youngsters hate to get shampoo suds and water streaming over their faces. My four-year-old niece, Pamela, has always been shampoo-shy. My sister, Marianne, solves this problem with a *shampoo shield*. Available through mail-order catalogs, a shampoo shield is a cushiony soft circular visorlike "cap" with a cutout crown that fits over your child's head. The watertight wide brim shields your little one's face so that you can shampoo and rinse her hair without getting any soapy water into her eyes, ears, and mouth.

Tip for easy sudsing: If you find it slippery business to hold your child with one hand and uncap and pour out the shampoo with the other, try this trick. Before bath time, transfer your baby shampoo into a flip-top bottle or empty liquid soap pump dispenser. (You may want to fix the bottle with a label that says "Baby Shampoo.") This simple strategy will make it easier for you to keep a firm grip on your little one while you measure out the shampoo you need.

You can continue to follow the shampooing steps described in chapter 2 well into the toddler years. By the time your child is three or four years old she may be ready to learn how to wash her own hair (always with adult supervision, of course).

At this age, your child can run her hands through the lather, but she still needs help, especially with rinsing. To make hair washing go smoothly, turn your shampoo lesson into a game. My mother had me pretend that I was a mermaid and would then pursuade me to "swim" under her "waterfall" so that she could wash and rinse my hair.

Another strategy: Step into the shower or tub with your child and demonstrate how you wash your own hair. (Little girls can shower or bathe with Mom, while little boys may prefer to be with Dad.) Then walk your child through her own lathering and rinsing steps, making sure the suds and water don't get into her eyes.

To help your child learn good hair care habits, it pays to brush up on the basics of gentle shampooing yourself. Use the following steps as a guide.

STEP-BY-STEP SHAMPOOING

1. Before lathering up, rinse hair thoroughly with comfortably warm water. Rinsing helps to dislodge dirt and grime and makes it easier to work up a good lather.
2. Pour a small amount of shampoo into your hand and massage palms together. Next, smooth your hands over the length of the hair.
3. Teach your child to use the pads of her fingertips to massage the shampoo into her scalp. Next, working from front to back, gently massage lather into hair. (Aggressive scrubbing can scratch the scalp and rough up the outer layer of the hair, making it prone to breakage.)
4. Although it seems like fun, do not pile hair on top of the head and wash it to and fro. This can cause tangling.
5. After a few minutes of thorough—and gentle—shampooing, rinse hair thoroughly with mildly warm water. Rinse hair for at least sixty seconds or longer, depending on hair length. A final rinse of cool water helps to tighten the cuticle for extra shine.
6. Gently blot hair with a clean dry towel. Do not rub! Brisk rubbing will cause snarls.

Once your child is about seven years old, he should be ready to shampoo his hair on his own. However, although he is independent enough to manage this task by himself (and most likely will not want you to have anything to do with it!), you may still have to keep after him to make sure that he does, indeed, wash his hair on a regular basis. (Youngsters at this age can be a little lackadaisical about grooming if left to their own devices!)

By the time your child is around the age of eleven or twelve, chances are she won't need any prodding to shampoo her hair. If anything, you will need to stock up on shampoo and remind your child not to wash her hair more than once a day.

SHAMPOO TIMETABLE

How often should you shampoo your child's hair? That depends. During baby's first year it is sufficient to wash her hair once or twice a week, according to many pediatricians. Once your child's hair is a bit longer, you may want to step up her shampooing schedule. To keep your child's hair clean and shining, try to shampoo her hair at least every other day.

Frequency of cleansing also depends on how active your child is. During the summer your child may often work up a healthy sweat while playing outdoors. Tucking hair under a snug hat in winter can also cause your child's scalp to perspire. In both instances, natural scalp oil can mix with dirt and perspiration, making your child's hair limp and lank. The solution: daily shampooing.

African-Americans' hair needs special care. Blacks tend to produce less sebum than Caucasians, so that dry scalp and dry hair can be a problem. Although Black hair is dry, it needs routine shampooing to wash away the buildup of dead, dry scales on the scalp and to keep the hair clean. To bring out the beauty of Black hair, your child's hair can be shampooed every two weeks or more frequently as needed.

SMOOTHING OUT TANGLES

If you follow the shampoo steps shown above, your child's hair shouldn't tangle too badly. However, you should still use TLC when combing wet hair. Water breaks the hydrogen bonds in the cortex that give hair its strength. Because wet hair is fragile, yanking a comb through tangles causes breakage and can hurt your child's scalp. For snarl-free combing, try these easy how-tos.

1. Spritz hair with a children's detangling spray. A detangling spray is a must for fine, curly, or kinky hair that tends to knot up after shampooing.

2. A wide-tooth comb glides through hair with a minimum of wear and tear. Opt for one made of rubber or wood. If you use a plastic comb, choose one with well-spaced teeth, and be sure that the tips on the teeth are smooth. Jagged tips can tear the hair and scratch the scalp.
3. Working on one section at a time, comb hair at the ends first, using downward strokes. When the knots are smoothed out, place the comb in the middle of the section of hair and gently comb through. Continue combing in this way, gradually working toward the roots. Last, when all hair is untangled, gently comb hair from roots to ends.
4. Never brush wet hair! Brushing stretches and weakens wet hair and can cause breakage.

CONDITIONING

You should begin to condition your child's hair as soon as it is more than four inches long. While a detangling rinse softens the hair and makes it easier to comb, a conditioner fills in the cracks of the cuticle brought on by brushing, combing, and everyday exposure to the elements. A conditioner also replenishes the hair's water supply and helps hair bounce back with more body and shine. To start, condition your child's hair once a week.

Gentle tear-free baby conditioners are available for babies and toddlers. For youngsters past the toddler stage there are mild hypoallergenic formulas for children. You can also dilute your own conditioner if you use a light rinse-out moisturizing conditioner meant for everyday use. Simply add a teaspoon of conditioner to eight ounces of mildly warm water.

How Much Is Enough?

A child's hair does not need heavy conditioning. In fact, too much conditioner can weigh down the hair, making it limp, lifeless, and a magnet for dirt and grime. A teaspoon, more or less, is a good gauge; hair past the shoulders will need more, enough to work through the length of the hair.

Your child's hair type also comes into play when measuring out conditioner. Fine hair needs less than hair of average thickness, and thick, coarse hair needs more.

Applying Conditioner

For mistake-proof conditioning, try the following simple Dos and Don'ts. When your child begins to shampoo her own hair, teach her these conditioning steps.

> **Don't** pour conditioner directly on the hair. Dousing hair with conditioner gives you too much of a good thing.
>
> **Do** measure out a small amount of conditioner into the palm of your hand, then massage your hands back and forth to disperse the conditioner.
>
> **Do** use a light hand to work conditioner through hair. To prevent split ends, be careful to apply conditioner to the ends, which are the oldest, most worn part of the hair.
>
> **Don't** leave conditioner on the hair for more than a minute. Thirty to sixty seconds is all it takes to condition a child's hair.
>
> **Do** rinse hair thoroughly with mildly warm water until water runs clear. To avoid tangling, rinse hair from front to back. Finish with a cool-water rinse.

YEAR-ROUND CARE FOR HEALTHY HAIR

Changes of the season bring on shifts in your child's hair care needs. A drop in the temperature or a rise in humidity can affect the way your child's hair behaves. As you read through this section you'll see how easy it is to cope with common hair hassles. And you'll get all the help you need in teaching your child good hair management skills!

Winter Woes

Cold, wind, and low humidity outdoors plus dry, hot air indoors and the overuse of blow-dryers can result in trouble for your child's hair. A dry, flaky scalp, limp locks, and flyaway hair are among the most common winter hair care problems. To the rescue, these easy solutions.

Stop static. When the air becomes cold and dry, hair loses moisture and its negative electrical charge builds up. As a result, individual strands begin to repel each other, making hair flyaway. Friction from brushing or combing the hair increases this static, because the bristles and teeth are also negatively charged. The positive charge of conditioner will neutralize hair's negative charge. Or try this instant static smoother: spritz a hairbrush with hair spray or an antistatic clothing spray. Spraying the inside of your child's winter hat will also help to keep flyaway hair under control.

Soothe dry scalp. Moisture loss due to low humidity and overuse of heat appliances such as blow-dryers can result in a dry, flaky scalp. While it may look a lot like dandruff, dry scalp should not be treated with dandruff shampoos. As a rule, children under twelve years of age do not have problems with dandruff, which is the result of overactive oil glands on the scalp. The itchiness and fine flaking of dry scalp are caused by a lack of water, not a buildup of oil. When skin cells on the scalp are low on water, they flake off. A moisturizing shampoo made for dry scalp will help to reduce flaking as it soothes itching.

Perk up flat hair. When the humidity drops, hair can go flat. And if you're shampooing less frequently during the cold weather months, hair will lose body. What helps to build body: routine washing with a gentle shampoo. When you condition your child's hair, try a light, oil-free rinse-out conditioner. It won't leave a sticky residue, which can weigh down hair.

Help for hat hair. Tucking your child's hair under a hat will keep her head warm but may mat hair down. Here's how to give hair a lift once your child is indoors. Take off the hat and lightly mist hair with plain tap water. (Try pouring the water in a plant mister for easy spraying.) Do not soak the hair; hair should be slightly damp, not wet. Then run your fingers through the hair, lifting hair up and away from the scalp.

HERE'S LOOKING AT YOU, KID!

Summer Survival

Hot, sticky weather can put your child's hair on its worst behavior. Curly hair can frizz up, while straight hair can go limp. Swimming and sunning can also take their toll on hair. For simple summer hair care solutions, read on.

Tame the frizzies. When the humidity is high, water in the atmosphere swells up the hair and softens the hydrogen bonds that hold the shape of the hair in place. This gives curly hair extra spring, but sometimes hair can get out of control. To smooth frizz, try a dab or two of one of the new antifrizz treatments, gel-like liquids formulated to limit hair's ability to absorb surface moisture. Can't find this treatment in your store? A quarter-size dollop of body lotion will do in a pinch. Rub the body lotion into your hands, then smooth palms over ends of clean, dry hair. This will also add shine.

Prevent sun damage. Overexposure to sunlight can rob hair of precious moisture. Too much sun can also burn the tender skin of your child's scalp. While your best defense against sun damage is to have your child wear a hat while playing outdoors, it may not always be practical. Stroking a sunscreen stick over the scalp where your child parts his hair or where hair is thin helps to burnproof the scalp. To counteract the drying effects of the sun, you can also spritz your child's tresses with a spray-on conditioning sunscreen for the hair. Another option: Philip Kingsley's Swimcap Cream, a water-repellent creamy hair conditioner with sunscreen made to be applied to hair before your child hits the water. Swimproof as well as sunproof, it protects the hair and scalp, and helps to minimize tangles after swimming.

R_x for chlorine damage. Even if your child wears a bathing cap when swimming in a chlorinated pool, hair can take a beating. Chlorine saps water from the hair, making it coarse and brittle. The copper ions in swimming pool disinfectants can also give blond hair a greenish cast. The cure: after your child's dip in the pool, rinse hair immediately. Once you're home, wash your child's hair with a deep-cleansing shampoo made to dislodge chlorine deposits. This formula converts chlorine into water-soluble chlorides, which are then easily rinsed away. For the best results, shampoo hair as soon as possible.

TLC for saltwater damage. Salt water robs hair of moisture, making hair brittle and prone to breakage. After a day at the beach, rinse hair with fresh water, then comb a light conditioner through the hair. Spray-on formulas are easy to tote in your beach bag. Once you're home, shampoo your child's hair with a gentle conditioning shampoo.

RESCUES FOR HAIR AND SCALP PROBLEMS

Of course, there are some problems that you can't solve simply by washing them away. They can be minor headaches such as getting chewing gum out of your child's hair, or they can be more serious and require prompt medical attention. Herewith, a roundup of safe, sure solutions for common hair and scalp problems.

Fast Fix for Getting Out Gum

When your child comes to you with a wad of chewing gum in her hair, don't attempt to snip it off with scissors—you'll wreak havoc with the shape of her haircut. A better way to cope with this sticky situation: Place an ice cube over the gummed-up section of hair for a few minutes. This freezes the gum so that it will easily peel off. If the gum continues to stick, apply a small amount of baby oil, then use fingers to slide off the gum. A little lemon juice mixed with water will dissolve the baby oil. Another option: massage a dollop of peanut butter into hair, then gently comb out gum. Olive oil or a dab of your cold cream will also do the trick. Be sure to shampoo your child's hair after one of these treatments!

Help for Head Lice

If your child comes home from school with an especially itchy scalp or is constantly scratching his head, check for head lice. Your child's grooming habits may be impeccable; however, three to five elementary schoolchildren out of every one hundred are infected with head lice, no matter what their social and economic background. While not a problem for Black children, head lice tend to affect primarily Caucasian schoolchildren. At first glance, a head lice infestation looks like dandruff. What appear to be white flakes are actually the white, oval-shaped nits (eggs) clinging to the shafts of hair. The nits are stubborn and cannot be brushed out of the hair.

Much more difficult to detect are the adult lice, which are about the size of sesame seeds and nest on the scalp. Because head lice are hard to see, you need to examine your child's hair and scalp under a bright light. Be sure to check areas around the ears, neck, back of scalp, and the hairline around the face. If your child has been scratching his head because of the intense itching, you may find scratch marks on the scalp. Check carefully, since open scratches can lead to a secondary infection. Should your child, indeed, have head lice, a doctor's visit is in order. While the most widely prescribed treatment is a medicated shampoo containing lindane, the safety of this ingredient for young children has been called into question. Safer alternatives include preparations formulated with pyrethrins, benzyl benzoate, and sulfur.

Before shampooing your child's hair, dislodge the nits with a fine-tooth comb. Gently wash your child's hair—and be sure to rinse out every trace of shampoo. *Note:* Since the shampoo is a medication, do not allow your child to wash his own hair. This lessens the chances of getting shampoo in the eyes or mouth. Repeat the treatment ten days later.

To safeguard the rest of your family, check every member's hair and scalp. (Adults can get head lice, too!) Launder clothes and bed linen in hot water, and run your clothes dryer on the hot cycle.

To avoid future infestation, tell your children not to share personal belongings such as combs, scarves, caps, and bed linen. You may want to speak to other parents and teachers to make sure that all affected children in your child's school are treated. Because of the social stigma attached to the problem of head lice, it is important that you remain calm. Treat your child's condition gently and matter-of-factly. This will help to take the pressure off, and to make what is a nuisance for both you and your child easier to handle.

Cure for Ringworm

Children between the ages of two and ten are susceptible to ringworm, a fungal infection of the scalp. The symptoms are patches of scales in a round shape or ring. The ring may be the size of a quarter and be pink in the center. The hair growing out of the scaly patch is usually thin and broken.

Unless it is treated promptly, ringworm can spread over your child's head and to other areas of the body. Children can also pass it on to each other. The treatment: oral antifungal medication as prescribed by a dermatologist. After six weeks of treatment, symptoms should disappear. By puberty children are less vulnerable to ringworm. One theory has it that during adolescence fatty acids in the scalp develop and may help to fight off this infection.

Coping with Hair Loss

Out of the blue your child may develop a patchy hair loss. Seeing bald spots where previously your child's hair had been healthy is a distressing and bewildering experience. The medical term for this condition is *alopecia areata*, and it is the result of an autoimmune function of the body. This type of hair loss is sometimes associated with diseases such as diabetes, conditions such as pernicious anemia, or an underactive thyroid. However, your child can develop alopecia areata without having any of these conditions. Sometimes an accident or emotional trauma can trigger this hair loss.

The good news is that this condition is simple to treat. Your dermatologist can give your child injections of steroids, which promote hair growth. If you're concerned with giving your child steroids, you may choose to forgo this treatment. Within three months your child's hair should grow back by itself. In the meantime, treat your child's hair and scalp tenderly and reassure her that the problem is temporary and will go away. If you suspect that emotional trauma has caused this condition, be sure to give your child the care and attention she needs.

Sometimes patches of short, fine little hairs may be a sign that your child has been pulling out his hair. In this case a child is, indeed, experiencing trauma, bottling up emotion, and is literally tearing out his hair in frustration. In this case, you may want to seek professional counseling for your child. Behavioral therapy can help your child to open up and express the thoughts and feelings that are troubling him. If your child is too young for therapy, give him extra doses of tender loving care at home. Your own attentiveness and concern may be all your child needs to solve this problem.

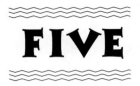

FIVE

Hair Shape-up: How to Cut, Curl, and Style Your Child's Hair

"**W**HAT'S THE BEST way to trim my toddler's bangs?" "Is blow-drying bad for my child's hair?" "Can I give my little girl a perm?" "Help! How can I brush the knots out of my child's hair?" "How can I tame a stubborn cowlick?"

These are a few of the questions that inevitably pop up when I talk to moms and dads about hair care for their kids. (Do they sound familiar?) Like you, they want their children's hair to behave beautifully and yet still look soft and natural—and with a minimum of fuss.

While some kids could care less about the way their hair is cut and styled, others have very strong feelings on the subject. After starting preschool, my young friend Dallas, then three years old, insisted on having his blond hair clipped short with a ducktail trailing down his neck! My brothers all hated their childhood crew cuts, and at age five, I was mortified whenever my mother cut my bangs too short. (My mother, of course, thought I looked adorable.)

Why does the way your child's hair looks become such an emotionally charged issue? Because neatness counts, because when it comes to good looks, hair is the "mane attraction." Somehow, pressed clothes, polished shoes, and clean fingernails can't make up for unruly hair.

At the same time, you want your child to feel comfortable and to feel good about the way his hair looks. As your child grows up, he becomes aware that his hair sends loud and clear signals about how he sees himself and wants others to see him.

This chapter is for every parent who has tried to cut, comb, and coax a child's hair into place, and who wants more coaching on how to perfect everyday hair care skills.

You'll learn how to baby your infant's hair. You'll get the scoop on how to take the trauma out of trimming your child's hair plus a step-by-step guide to cutting hair like a pro. This chapter also offers a crash course in blow-drying basics, styling safety tips, advice on whether to perm or straighten your child's hair, and more.

Caring for your child's hair should be a breeze, not a battle. The more both of you enjoy it, the easier it will become for your child to make good hair care a habit.

SPECIAL CARE FOR BABY'S HAIR

Should you brush your infant's hair during her first year of life? As long as you're gentle, the answer is yes. Brushing massages the scalp, increasing the flow of blood that carries oxygen and nutrients to the hair follicles.

If you're worried about damaging the "soft spot" (fontanel) on a baby's head, relax. Nature protects it with a thick membrane. Just don't brush too vigorously. Aggressive brushing can irritate the scalp and weaken baby's hair. A few light, quick, short strokes will do nicely.

Be sure to use a baby brush with fine, silky bristles. A natural bristle brush is best. To check for gentleness, run the brush over your cheek. If the brush feels scratchy or the bristles don't bend, toss it.

Some hair care experts prefer a comb over a brush, since a comb puts less stress on the hair and scalp. If you do opt for a baby comb, make sure the teeth have soft, blunt tips. Sharp teeth can snag baby's hair and scratch the scalp.

ACCESSORY ALERT

If you're the parent of a baby girl, you may find it tempting to dress up her hair with a pretty clip or fancy bow. Don't. It's too easy for your baby to pull the ornament out of her hair and swallow it. The best way to keep your little one's hair out of her eyes is to keep it trimmed. There will be plenty of time during childhood to play with hair accessories later on.

Giving Tangles the Brush

"My daughter won't let me brush the knots out of her hair. It's always a tangled mess! What can I do?"

More than one mother has asked me to help her with this problem. If you follow the post-shampoo detangling tips in chapter 4, your child's hair shouldn't knot up as badly. But during the course of a child's rough-and-tumble day, it's easy for fine or curly hair to become tangled.

To *smooth out* tangles, use a small brush with wide-spaced, bendable nylon or plastic bristles with smooth tips. (Natural bristles are too soft to penetrate knots.) Brushing one section of hair at a time, always start at the ends. (Trying to detangle hair from roots to ends puts too much tension on the scalp.) Gently grasp the ends of each section in your free hand as you brush out the tangles with short strokes.

If your child simply won't let you brush out all her tangles, don't try to push her. This will only result in her growing to dislike and avoid brushing her hair.

I always tell parents that their children may be more cooperative if they make a hair-brushing session more enticing. If you say, "Let's make your hair pretty," or "Why don't we make your hair soft and shiny?" your child may be less reluctant than if you were to say, "I want to brush out all those messy knots in your hair," which sounds painful. Accentuating the positive isn't like waving a magic wand, but it's well worth a try.

CUTTING HAIR: TEAR-FREE TRIMS FOR KIDS

The way your child's hair behaves and falls into line depends on having a good haircut. However, given the expense of each trip to the barber shop or hair salon, regular haircuts can add up to be hard on your wallet.

To trim the high cost of professional cuts, you may want to take on the task at home between salon visits. One advantage: your child may feel more secure in familiar surroundings. Another: your child may be more willing to sit still for you rather than a stranger.

When my brother Bobby was three years old, my dad took him along to the barber shop. Bobby watched intently as the barber snipped, combed, and fussed over my dad's hair. But once my dad was ready to leave the shop, Bobby burst into tears. He wanted *his* hair cut, too! In seconds he was propped up in the chair and swathed in an oversize cape as the barber obligingly faked a few quick clips along the back of my brother's head. Bobby was all smiles.

My dad likes to tell this story because it runs counter to the more harrowing experiences he's had with his children's haircuts. More than once, each of my brothers had to be held down while a brave, good-hearted relative carefully snipped away. You're sure to have more luck—and better results—if you follow these simple dos and don'ts.

> **Do** trim your child's hair when he's relaxed and his energy level is low.
>
> **Don't** mention the word "cut." To a small child (especially a toddler) this can sound frightening. You're more likely to gain your child's confidence if you say, "Let's make you look handsome," or "Why don't we try a new style?"
>
> **Do** try to distract and relax your child. Work slowly. Talk as you trim. If you're cutting hair outdoors, call attention to what's going on in the backyard. If you're indoors, park your child in front of a mirror so he can watch what you're doing.
>
> **Don't** tug on your child's hair. Try to hold it gently between your fingers.

Hair Shape-up

Do keep your free hand between the scissors and your child's head to prevent accidents due to sudden movements. If possible, have another adult lightly but firmly hold your child's head.

Don't take longer than fifteen minutes tops. Your child's patience—and your own—has its limits!

Basic Equipment

To cut hair like a pro, you'll need the following:

- A pair of thin, straight, stainless steel scissors, about four to five inches long. Some experts recommend using shears with rounded tips. Check drugstores and hardware stores as well as stores that carry sewing and beauty supplies. Optional for cutting boys' hair: good hair clippers.
- A wide-tooth comb for smoothing out tangles and parting hair into sections.
- A plant mister or spray bottle filled with mildly warm water to dampen hair as you cut. (If your child's hair is curly or tends to knot up, add a small amount of cream rinse to the water.)
- A clean towel to drape around your child's neck and shoulders. (This keeps snippets of hair from collecting on your child's neck, which can make skin itchy.) Fasten ends together with a safety pin.
- A large, fluffy makeup brush (the kind used for applying loose powder) and a child's formula body powder. Dip the brush into a little powder poured into the palm of your hand and lightly dust loose hairs off your child's neck as you cut.

Setting Up Shop

The perfect spot for cutting your child's hair is an open, well-lit area. If possible, go outdoors. When you cut hair in your backyard or out on the deck, you don't have to worry about loose clippings getting into your carpeting or furnishings. Indoors, your bathroom doubles as a full-service salon. You have your sink for wetting hair, a mirror for watching your progress, a countertop or shelf for your equipment, adequate lighting, and an easy-to-sweep floor.

If your bathroom doesn't give you enough elbow room, try the rec room in your basement. Avoid cutting hair in your kitchen. You don't want stray hairs to be floating into areas where you prepare and cook your family's food!

You'll also need a chair or stool that's high enough to make it comfortable for you to cut your child's hair as he sits up straight. *Hint:* You might find wielding your shears is easier and less stressful for your youngster if you also sit down while you snip. Whether you choose to sit or stand, you need to feel relaxed and to have freedom of movement.

STEP-BY-STEP BASIC CUTS FOR BOYS AND GIRLS

Given a child's short attention span, and the fact that you probably did not graduate from beauty school, no one expects you to design a trendy new hairstyle for your child. But with a little know-how you *can* learn to trim bangs, clean up straggly ends, neaten sideburns, and spruce up the shape of an overgrown cut. Even if you're all thumbs, you'll find it easy to follow the step-by-step instructions for children's haircuts coming up. All are low-maintenance, wash-and-wear styles designed by expert hairstylist Glen Davis of Nubest & Co. Salon in Manhasset, New York.

In most cases, your child's hair will be easier to cut if it's just been shampooed and conditioned. If this is not practical, spritz hair with mildly warm water. Lightly rewet hair as it dries. Note that curly and wavy hair shrinks as it dries, so trim less of this hair than you think you need to.

One last tip: to make cutting easier, begin on your right side if you're right-handed; on your left side if you're a lefty. And try to keep your child's head erect. Now you're ready to begin!

Hair Shape-up

STRAIGHT-TO-WAVY SHORT CUT FOR BOYS AND GIRLS

1. Comb damp hair back, then push forward. Next, comb hair on sides straight out from temples. Combing hair in one-inch to two-inch-wide sections, hold each section between fingers and trim straight across. Hair should be softly fringed when combed flat.

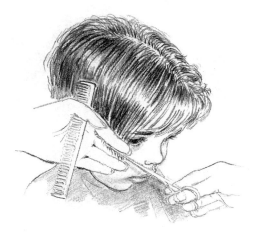

2. To get sideburns even, choose a spot close to where the earlobe meets the head. This will act as your guide for sideburn length. Use the same spot for both sideburns and adjust the length accordingly.

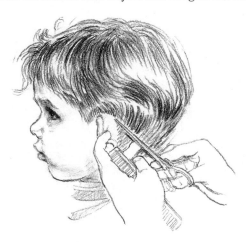

3. In back, comb hair straight out from the skull. Starting with the top layer, take one-inch- to two-inch-wide sections. Following curve of head, trim hair straight across using length at sides as guide.

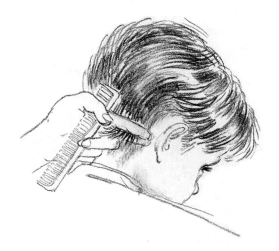

4. In front, comb hair up and forward so that it comes to a point. Hold away from face and trim ends. Again, this method works whether your child has bangs or side-parts his hair.

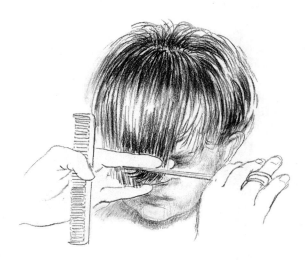

Hair Shape-up

5. The easy-care finish: allow hair to dry naturally or lightly blow-dry.

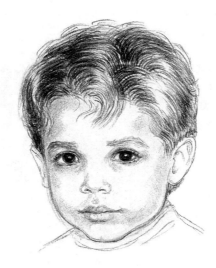

BASIC BOY'S CUT FOR BLACK HAIR

1. Hair cutting will go more quickly if you cut your son's hair dry. Simply fluff hair out with a wide-tooth comb or pick.

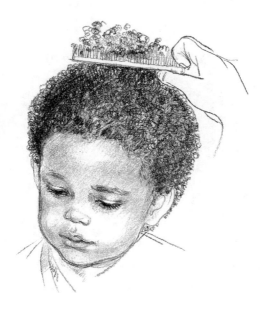

HERE'S LOOKING AT YOU, KID!

2. Using hair clippers, trim hair short at hairline, slightly curving outward and ending above temples. The longest length of hair should be 1½ to 3 inches long.

3. Clip crown to desired length following curve of head. Next, trim from each side toward the back; then, trim the back following curve of head. Blend top and sides by rounding corners of top.

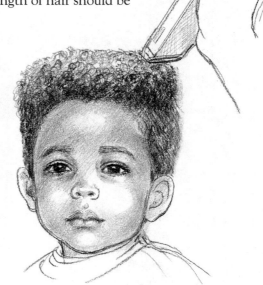

4. The neat results: dampen hair and work in a little leave-in conditioner. Gently pat hair into place with hands.

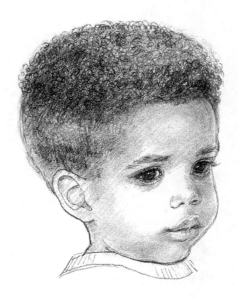

SHOULDER-LENGTH BLUNT CUT FOR GIRLS

1. Starting in back, part damp hair down the center. At ear level, divide each side and either comb the top sections forward over ears or clip into place. This gives you a top layer on both sides of the center part and a bottom layer.

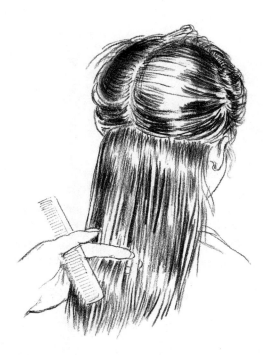

2. Holding your scissors and comb in one hand, take a one-inch- to two-inch-wide section of hair in your free hand. Comb the section straight down, gently sliding fingers of free hand down as you comb. Stop just above the point that you want to trim.

3. Holding the section taut between your middle and index fingers, shift the comb into your free hand. Snip hair that shows below fingers. Continue this pattern until the bottom layer is trimmed.

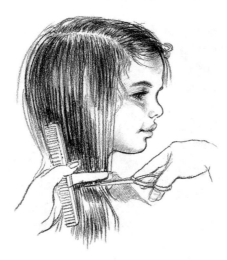

4. Next, unclip or free the top layer and comb it straight down. One section at a time, hold hair between fingers and trim hair straight across. Then tilt your child's head forward, comb hair flat against neck, and snip the stray hairs that show beneath the solid line of hair. (Retrimming hair allows ends to curve under.)

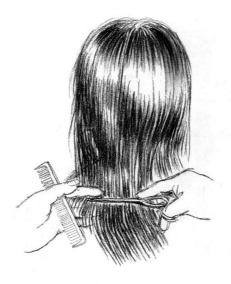

Hair Shape-up

5. To trim the right side, part your child's hair off-center on the left. Turn her head to the left and tilt it away from you. One section at a time, trim side even with chin line. To trim the left side, part your child's hair off-center on the right. Turn your child's head to the right. Again, with the head tilted away from you, trim side even with chin line. This method helps to balance the weight of the hair.

6. To check for evenness, pull pieces at sides forward. Simply take a one-inch-wide section in front of ears. Comb hair on either side of ears forward to meet at chin. Trim as needed.

7. To trim bangs, comb hair that falls in front of hairline at temples into a triangular section above eyes and lift about three inches away from the bridge of the nose. Cut a *small* amount. If hair is wavy or curly, allow an extra one-fourth to one-half inch for hair to shrink up. Check to see that bangs are the length you want. Repeat trimming as needed. This method layers bangs to lighten the weight.

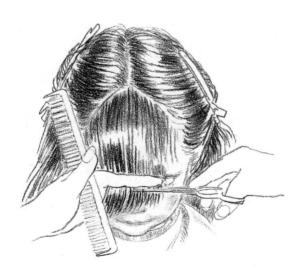

8. A classic cut shows off shiny hair and is less apt to tangle.

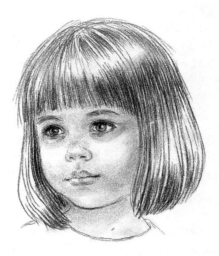

BASIC GIRL'S CUT FOR BLACK HAIR

1. Comb through damp hair with a wide-tooth comb. Next, comb hair in front of ears forward.

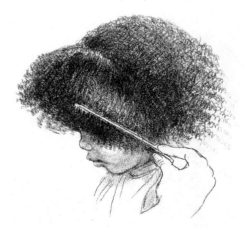

2. Working on one side at a time, start in front and tilt scissors on a deep 45-degree angle. Separating one-inch-wide sections with your comb, hold section between middle and index fingers of free hand. Snip ends between fingers. Trim each side on an angle so that it is shortest in front, gradually becoming longer to blend in an oval shape with the hair in back.

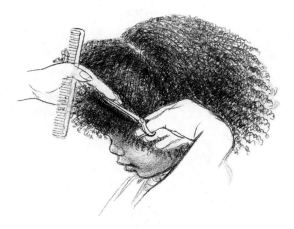

3. Comb hair straight down in back. Working along the bottom, take one-inch-wide sections with your comb, hold hair between fingers, and trim ends below fingers straight across. Repeat until the hair along the bottom is trimmed. Use the bottom of the angle of hair at the sides as your guide for the proper length.

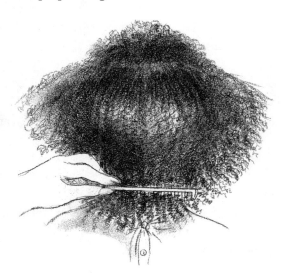

4. Short and sassy. Apply a leave-in conditioner or conditioning oil and style hair with fingertips.

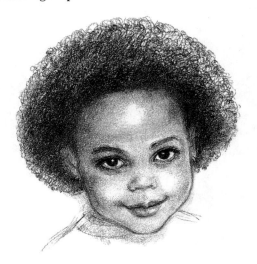

BLOW-DRYING BASICS

A blow dryer is a great hair care time-saver. However, it does take a little skill to use properly. To simplify your life, you may want to let your child's hair dry naturally whenever possible. Simply towel-dry and comb hair into place.

Babies and toddlers certainly don't need to have their hair blown dry! Baby hair is so fine that any moisture will evaporate in minutes. But around age three or four a child's hair becomes thicker and takes longer to dry; there may be days when you'll want to take some hair care shortcuts.

Will blow-drying damage your child's hair? No, as long as you don't overdo it. (Hair actually cools down as water evaporates.) To make blow-drying gentle on your child's hair, follow these simple dos and don'ts.

> **Do** use a clean, dry towel to gently blot excess moisture from your child's hair before blow-drying. Hair should be damp, not wet.
>
> **Do** lightly spritz your child's hair with a leave-in conditioner or a special treatment meant to protect hair against heat from styling appliances.

Hair Shape-up

Do set your blow dryer's heat setting on medium. The cool setting is too chilly for most kids. (And hair drying will take longer.) The hot setting will overheat and dry out hair and may burn the scalp. Adjust the air-flow speed to low rather than high.

Don't hold the dryer too close to your child's hair. Keep it at least six to eight inches away.

Don't concentrate warm blasts of air on any one section of the hair at any time. Keep the dryer moving up and down the length of the hair.

Do turn off your dryer while your child's hair is still slightly damp and allow it to dry naturally. This prevents frizzies.

TO PERM OR NOT TO PERM

A halo of frothy curls certainly has its charms. But if your daughter was born with straight hair and your heart is set on her having curls, you may want to give her a perm. Don't.

To put curl in straight hair, the chemical bonds that hold the protein molecules of the hair in place must be broken with a strong alkaline waving solution. This might be fine for an adult's hair, but it is hard on a child's delicate hair.

The perming process dehydrates the hair. As a result, chemically treated tresses are more fragile and prone to breakage than untreated hair. Granted, today's perm formulas are gentler than the kits that were available when you were growing up. But they still must be potent enough to *break* the bonds of the hair. The chemicals may also cause your child's scalp to flare up and can irritate any abrasions or cuts.

There are other important reasons why it may not be a good idea to have a young child's hair permed. Trying to change the curl pattern of your daughter's hair may also take away from her sense that her hair is just fine the way it is, thank you. Feeling that she needs waves or curls in order to conform to a "look" or a trend or to please Mom and Dad can be rough on a child's self-esteem. Knowing that you take pleasure in what her hair does naturally will bring your daughter a step closer to a positive self-image.

MAKING WAVES

Of course, if your child *wants* to have curly or wavy hair now and then—it can be fun to change and play with what hair can do—there are alternatives that are kinder to the hair and scalp. The following easy sets are a snap to do—and sure to be big hits with the pajama party crowd!

Wrap-and-Tie Set

Michael Gordon, owner of Bumble & Bumble Salon in New York City, suggests setting your daughter's hair with snippets of cotton gauze or cheesecloth. This fresh take on the old-fashioned rag set works best for medium-length hair (from chin length to above the shoulders).

Cut the cloth into strips that are one to two inches wide and six to seven inches long. Mist your child's hair with mildly warm water or a detangling spray.

Starting in front, part hair into one-inch-wide sections. One at a time, take a section and place it in the middle of a strip of cloth. Wrap hair around the cloth as you twist it toward the scalp. Take the ends of the cloth and tie in a secure (but not tight) knot.

When your child's hair is dry, undo the knots and remove the cloth wraps. Have your child shake her head to loosen her new curls. Next, as your daughter bends from the waist, lift her hair lightly from underneath with a wide-tooth comb. When your daughter tosses her hair back, her hair will be a tumble of light, airy waves and curls.

Roll-and-Bend Set

If your daughter's hair is long, try setting it on flexible, cushiony soft styling rods, available at drugstores and beauty supply shops. The soft rods don't pull on the scalp as tightly as conventional rollers. And you don't need pins or clips to hold the rod in place.

To start, lightly mist hair with mildly warm water or detangling spray. Starting in front, take a one-inch to two-inch-wide section of hair and place a rod at the bottom. Roll hair on the rod toward the scalp, then bend the ends into a **C** shape. This secures the rod. Once hair is dry, undo the rods and follow the shake-and-comb styling steps described in the wrap-and-tie set (page 106).

Perfect Pincurl Set

To put waves and curls in short hair, try a simple pincurl set. Start in front and work toward the back. Alternating rows, wind one row clockwise, the next counterclockwise.

Mist your child's hair with mildly warm water or a detangling spray. Starting at the roots, make one-inch-wide sections. Wind each section around one or two fingers. Slip the curled hair off your finger, tuck the loose end under, and secure with a bobby pin. Bobby pins should have protective rubber tips. Do not open pins with your teeth; this could break off the tips.

Once hair is dry, undo pincurls. Follow the shake-and-comb styling steps from the wrap-and-tie set.

STYLING TLC FOR BLACK HAIR

To show off the beauty and texture of Black hair, treat it kindly. Perhaps you like to braid your child's hair into carefree cornrows. While it is a becoming style, braiding your child's hair too tightly can hurt her scalp and damage her hair. The constant pulling and tugging are hard on the hair follicles. When hair is in constant traction, the hair bulb is stretched. Eventually, the hair breaks off or falls out.

For a gentler approach to corn-rowing, try these hair care tips from Turning Heads Salon in New York City, a salon that specializes in care for Black hair.

- Braid hair loosely—do not pull on the scalp. It is especially important to reduce tension at the hairline, where hair can break off.
- Consider redoing cornrows every few days. This is better for your child's hair than braiding it tightly for the sake of having a long-lasting style.

- Every few days dab the parts between cornrows with fresh cotton moistened with witch hazel or an herbal toner. This helps to keep the scalp clean.
- Your child can sleep on cornrows. Just be sure to remove any beads or barrettes before she goes to bed.
- Do not let your child wear cornrows for more than two or three weeks at a time. Her hair and scalp need a chance to relax!
- Be sure to shampoo your child's hair at least once a week, even with cornrows intact.

Straight Talk about Straightening

Should you straighten a young child's hair? In my opinion, no. Hair straightening (or relaxing) works in the same way as a perm does to break the bonds of the hair. A strong relaxing solution is applied to the hair and then the curls are combed out. Like a perm, a relaxing treatment dries out the hair and leaves it in a more fragile state. The solution also has to be applied close to the roots of the hair, which can irritate the scalp.

There are now special hair relaxing kits for children ages five and up. The relaxing solution in these kits is formulated without lye, which is said to make the formula milder. However, it is recommended that the health of your child's hair be checked first with a professional analysis. And for upkeep, your child's hair would have to be touched up every six to eight weeks. To me, that sounds like more trouble than it's worth. Keeping your child's hair healthy and in good condition is more important.

A neat haircut, soft braids and ponytails, and loose cornrows are all good styling options for your child's hair. To play up the natural texture of your child's hair, comb in a leave-in conditioner or hair oil made with herbal and plant extracts. They absorb into the hair, give it a gloss, and protect the scalp without clogging pores. Do not use pomades. They are made with mineral oil and wax, which just sit on top of the hair and dry it out. Eventually this causes breakage.

STYLING TIPS AND TRICKS

When it comes to fixing your child's hair, less is more. That is, less fuss gives more natural-looking results. Less tugging and pulling means more damage control and healthier hair. Whether your goal is simply to keep your child's hair out of her eyes, or to add a stylish accent, the following tips will help.

Cures for Cowlicks

There's more than one way to lick a cowlick. This is, as I'm sure you know, a stubborn piece of hair that sticks up because it grows out of the scalp in different directions; cowlicks usually show up in the front.

Allowing your child's hair to grow longer in this area is one solution. The weight of longer hair helps the cowlick to lie flat. In the meantime, you can tame an unruly cowlick when you blow-dry your child's hair. Apply a dab of styling gel or hair sculpting lotion. Catch the end of the cowlick with a styling brush, pull it straight, and blow-dry.

Or try the art of the part: either part your child's hair through the middle of the cowlick, or make a part alongside it.

Accents on Accessories

Barrettes, headbands, and ponytail holders are the extra added attractions that give you pretty ways to sweep your daughter's hair off her face. However, any accessory that holds the hair too tightly puts too much stress on the hair and scalp. To minimize pulling and tearing, follow these simple dos and don'ts.

> **Do** use coated elastic bands rather than plain rubber bands when you put your daughter's hair in a ponytail or braids. Rubber bands can snag and tear the hair.
> **Don't** make tight ponytails or braids. The tension on the scalp can result in hair loss along the hairline in front, a bald spot called *traction alopecia*.

Do change the placement of barrettes from day to day. This way you don't put tension on the same spot time after time.

Don't use hair combs unless your child's hair is thick enough to hold them. Combs usually slip out of a child's fine-textured hair.

Don't use headbands with sharp teeth that can scratch the scalp. Opt for stretchy fabric headbands.

Best Bets for Boys

Many of the preschool and school-age boys I know are surprisingly style-conscious. Having spiked-up or slicked-back "hip" hair goes with wearing rolled-up jeans and high-top sneakers. Kids are more likely to get their ideas about hairstyles from music videos, movies, or older siblings than from you. What's a parent to do? Try these easy ways to give your son's hair the latest style!

- To spike up a short haircut, comb a little mousse into clean, damp hair. Lift hair straight up with fingers. Then blow-dry hair with your dryer set on a low-speed setting. Or use a diffuser.
- Create a trendy grooved look. Simply comb a quarter-size dab of mousse through clean, damp hair with a wide-tooth comb. Let hair dry naturally.
- For nonsticky slicked-back hair, spritz a fine-tooth comb with a light spray gel. Comb clean, damp hair straight back. Let hair dry naturally.
- Show off the texture of curly or wavy hair. Rub a little liquid styling gel into clean, damp hair. Scrunch curls or waves with fingers. Blow-dry hair using a dryer with a diffuser attachment. Or allow hair to dry naturally.

Whether cutting or styling your child's hair, keep in mind that boys and girls alike link the way their hair looks with their self-image. A child as young as a preschooler knows that a haircut, like a favorite dress or T-shirt, expresses personal identity. While you will be in charge of what's neat and attractive for your child—at least until the preteen years—a little give-and-take will help your child to feel more self-assured and more comfortable with his appearance.

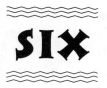

SIX

Smile! Dental Care for Your Child's Teeth and Gums

THE FIRST TIME your baby breaks into a smile, you're bedazzled. As your child grows up, his winning grin will tell people that he's confident, upbeat, open, and direct.

Not only do you want to keep your child's smile beautiful, you also want to keep it healthy. Thanks to good dental care and the efforts of parents just like you, half of America's children today are cavity free. If you want your child to be counted in this group, read on!

This chapter will take you through all the steps essential to proper care of your child's teeth and gums. You'll learn how to safeguard your child's smile *before* she cuts her first tooth, how to cope with the traumas of teething, and what to do if your child's tooth is knocked out.

Your child depends on you to teach him the right way to brush and floss. Learning the basics of dental hygiene *before* the first visit from the tooth fairy will give your child a definite edge in fighting tooth decay and gum disease.

But suppose you have a fussy toddler who won't brush, or who is afraid to go to the dentist. How can you be sure your child is getting enough fluoride to build strong, cavity-resistant teeth? Did you know that starchy foods are as bad for your child's teeth as sugary snacks?

HERE'S LOOKING AT YOU, KID!

How do you know whether or not your child will need braces? How long does it take to straighten a crooked smile, and what does it cost?

What you learn today will help your child to develop the good dental care habits that will keep his grin happy and healthy for a lifetime. And taking care of your child's teeth today will pay off with fewer and lower dental bills later. Now that's something to smile about!

KEEPING BABY'S SMILE SAFE

To get your baby's smile off to a healthy start, Nature provides some help. The natural sucking movements your baby makes during breast-feeding or bottle-feeding give the tongue and other muscles in your baby's mouth a good workout. Keeping baby's oral muscles strong helps to maintain teeth in their proper places as each tooth erupts through the gums.

But to maximize her chances of developing trouble-free teeth and gums, the American Academy of Pediatric Dentistry recommends that you begin a program of daily cleaning starting the first day of baby's life. Even though her teeth haven't erupted, the massaging action of cleaning will stimulate her gums. Then by the time your baby is five or six months old and cutting her first tooth, both you and your baby will be accustomed to a regular routine of dental care.

Regular cleaning keeps food residue and bacteria from harming your baby's teeth as they erupt. Plaque, a sticky, nearly colorless film, constantly forms on the teeth. If bacteria in the plaque build up on baby's teeth, they can lead to decay.

Why protect your child's baby teeth if they are only going to fall out later? Your child needs all twenty of his primary teeth to help him eat properly, speak clearly, and, of course, look his best. Baby teeth reserve space in the jaw for your child's permanent teeth. And having a full set of primary teeth allows your child's jaw and facial bones to develop properly. To make cleaning pleasant and easy for you and your baby, follow these simple steps.

CLEANING HOW-TOS

- Plan to clean your baby's mouth after every feeding and at bedtime.

- Make yourself and your baby comfortable. Sit in an easy chair or on the sofa and place your baby on her back with her head in your lap. Or lay your baby on a soft blanket on the floor or on the changing table. Whatever position you choose, be sure that it's easy to see into your infant's mouth.
- Take a fresh, damp gauze pad, or the corner of a clean, moistened washcloth. Then gently wipe your baby's mouth, gums, tongue, and any teeth that are coming in. Lightly massage the gums.
- Another option: in the morning and at bedtime rub baby's gums and teeth with Baby Oragel Tooth and Gum Cleanser, a special antibacterial gel tooth and gum cleanser. The sugar-free, fresh-tasting gel not only removes plaque but also helps to minimize plaque buildup.

Your Baby's First Teeth

Just as babies begin to walk and talk at varying ages, so it goes with teething. As a rule, your child's first tooth erupts around the age of six months. If your baby doesn't have her first tooth by her first birthday, consult a pediatric dentist. Once your child is three years old, you should be able to count a full set of twenty primary teeth in her mouth.

As soon as your child gets his first tooth, you should make an appointment with a pediatric dentist for his first dental checkup. The sooner your baby receives professional care, the better his chances for excellent dental health.

If you need assistance in locating a specialist in pediatric dentistry, contact the American Academy of Pediatric Dentistry for a list of referrals. Write: The American Academy of Pediatric Dentistry, 211 E. Chicago Ave., Suite 1036, Chicago IL 60611.

It is also best to make brushing baby's teeth routine as soon as the first tooth shows up, and definitely by the time he has six to eight primary teeth (between the ages of twelve to eighteen months). Areas of the gums that have no teeth should still be cleansed and massaged. And when all the primary teeth have erupted (usually by 2½ to 3 years of age), you can begin to floss your child's teeth.

Soothing Teething Pain

As you clean your baby's mouth, be sure to check her gums. If they are red and puffy, or you can see or feel the tip of a tooth emerging, chances are that your baby is teething. Other symptoms of teething are excessive drooling and cranky behavior. Your baby may also lose her appetite, change her eating habits, or have trouble sleeping.

Why can teething be so painful for your baby? When your little one's teeth are ready to cut through her gums, the soft tissue of the gums tends to swell and become tender. To ease baby's discomfort, try these easy soothers.

- Several times a day, wipe your baby's gums with a clean, damp gauze pad. Or gently massage her gums with a soft-bristle child's toothbrush.
- Give your baby something to chew on. A piece of toast may do the trick. Or try a teething ring made of firm rubber. *Do not use the type of teether meant to be frozen*—it may become too hard for baby's gums.
- Gently massage baby's gums with a clean finger. A small spoon cooled in the fridge may also offer some relief. You might also want to apply a teething gel such as Baby Oragel Teething Gel.
- During the toddler stage, when your child is cutting his molars, it may be tricky to apply a teething gel with your fingers. One solution comes from a *Parents* reader who wrote to us with this suggestion: Put a dab of anesthetic gel on your child's toothbrush. Tell him that it will help his mouth to stop hurting. Supervise your child as he brushes the gel on his gums. This may be more relaxing and less intrusive than trying to probe around your toddler's mouth with your fingers!
- Another *Parents* reader shares this tip: Give your child chunky pieces of frozen fruit to suck on. Try freezing pieces of peaches, pears, apples, and bananas. Note: avoid using small round fruits such as grapes, as they are choking hazards for children under four years of age.

- If teething seems to be unbearable for your child, ask your pediatrician or pediatric dentist to prescribe a medicine that will temporarily numb your baby's gums.
- If your baby also has a rash, fever, or is vomiting, chances are that teething is not the cause of his misery. Call your pediatrician immediately.

One last word of comfort: Remember that teething is temporary and a natural part of your baby's growth and development. As soon as the tooth has broken through the gums, all symptoms disappear!

Baby-Bottle Tooth Decay

You are about to put your baby down for a nap or to sleep for the night. Or your baby is fussing in between feedings and you want to pacify her. In each case you give your baby a bottle filled with milk, formula, fruit juice, or other sweetened liquid. And as you feed your baby, she falls asleep as she drinks. Sounds harmless enough, doesn't it? Yet over time, this habit can lead to a serious dental condition known as "baby-bottle tooth decay" or "nursing decay." Babies who are breast-fed are also susceptible.

Milk (including breast milk), fruit juices, and other sweetened liquids contain sugar. The bacteria in plaque feed on these sugars and produce acids that attack tooth enamel.

When your baby is awake, saliva in the mouth helps to carry the liquid away from the teeth. But the flow of saliva slows down during sleep. This allows the sugary liquid to pool around your baby's teeth. As your baby dozes, the liquid has time to activate plaque. The acids in the plaque attack tooth enamel for at least twenty minutes. Eventually, tooth decay can occur.

Damage is done quickly. The upper front teeth decay fastest, then the upper and lower back teeth. Left untreated, all your baby's teeth can be destroyed. The good news is that it is quite easy to prevent baby-bottle tooth decay. Simply follow these guidelines.

- Be sure to clean your child's teeth and gums thoroughly after each feeding.

- Do not put your child to sleep with a bottle containing milk formula, fruit juice, or other sweetened liquid.
- If you need to give your baby a bottle between feedings, before a nap, or at bedtime, opt for cool water. Or you may choose to give her a clean pacifier.
- Check your child's medications, including vitamins. Many contain sugar; while a little sweetening "helps the medicine go down," it adds to your baby's sugar intake. If you medicate your baby frequently, clean her mouth with a clean damp gauze pad each time.
- Pediatric dentists recommend that you stop bottle-feeding and breast-feeding your baby by the time she is twelve months old. Early weaning will help to minimize the chances of tooth decay.

BRUSHING BASICS

When can your child take charge of brushing his teeth? He can usually go solo by the age of six; up until then your child needs your help. It is recommended that children brush their teeth after every meal and at bedtime.

Brushing Up on Brushes

For the best results, the right toothbrush counts. For babies and children alike, choose a child-size toothbrush. Be sure that the size and shape of the head make it easy to reach every tooth. One option: a child-size diamond-shaped head is designed to maneuver easily in small mouths. A brush with a handle that's angled like a dental instrument makes less work of brushing hard-to-reach areas such as back teeth. Opt for a brush with extra-soft nylon bristles. The tips should be polished and gently rounded. You may want to ask your pediatric dentist to recommend a brush for your child.

To help a small child look forward to tooth-brushing, you may want to try a brush designed with one of his favorite superheroes or cartoon characters. A neon-bright color may also help to put extra zing in his routine. There are also glittery brushes, and for youngsters ages six to twelve there are brushes that glow in the dark!

The cutoff date for tossing a toothbrush is generally every three months. However, because preschoolers tend to brush imperfectly and chew on the bristles, they tend to weaken the brush quickly. It's best to do a toothbrush inspection on a regular basis. Worn-out, frayed bristles can't do an efficient job of cleaning teeth and may scratch or injure a child's tender gums.

Brushing Baby's Teeth

When your child has his second birthday, he is old enough to hold a toothbrush fairly well and can start to brush his own teeth—with your supervision, of course. However, since tooth decay can strike earlier than the age of two, you need to begin a routine of regular brushing as soon as your child's baby teeth start to come in. The following how-tos will show you the easiest way to brush baby teeth.

- Wet your child's toothbrush, but do not apply toothpaste. Until your child is two or three years old and able to rinse his mouth properly, he is likely to swallow some of the toothpaste. When children under the age of six swallow fluoride toothpastes on a regular basis, their teeth can develop a whitish mottling called fluorosis. (For more details see pages 124–25.)
- Try to brush teeth in a set order that you follow each time. For example, brush the lower front teeth first, then the upper front teeth; next, the lower back teeth and upper back teeth. Be sure to brush the inner surfaces as well as the outer. Having an order to follow will make it easier to do thorough brushing.
- Brush a small area at a time. Place the brush horizontally against the teeth and gum, then gently "scrub" teeth back and forth. To brush the inner surface of the front teeth, hold the brush in a vertical position; lightly brush teeth with up-and-down strokes.

- Use a light hand. Gentle brushing is quite effective in dislodging food particles and breaking up plaque.

Toothbrushing Tips for Fussy Toddlers

A friend of mine was having a tough time getting her toddler to stand still while she brushed his teeth. To help her find a solution, I called Marvin Berman, D.D.S., a pediatric dentist who practices in Chicago. Dr. Berman's simple strategy may work for you, too!

- Sit behind your child and hug him close to you with one hand. This keeps him from squirming and pulling away. Your gentle hug will also help him to feel relaxed and secure.
- Next, tilt your child's head back and have him look up at you. Give your child his toothbrush, then hold his hand as you guide his brushing strokes. This will give your child a sense of being in control.
- Sing silly songs or recite nursery rhymes. Or make funny faces. (From your toddler's point of view, you're already upside down!) Having fun will make the time pass quickly.
- Brush the lower front teeth first, then the upper front teeth. Do the back teeth last. When you brush the back teeth, your toddler may be afraid of choking or gagging, and that's the end of your brushing session. You have a better chance of finishing the job if you start in front.

Brushing for Two- to Six-Year-Olds

When your child is around the age of two he is ready to learn how to brush his teeth by himself. Kids love to imitate their parents, so you may want to show off your own brushing skills first and then let him take his turn. Remember, until your child is about six or seven, he doesn't have the dexterity to handle brushing on his own. Once your child finishes brushing, give teeth another cleaning yourself, just in case he may have missed an area. Thoroughness counts!

At this point you can moisten the end of your child's toothbrush with a small amount (no bigger than a pea) of fluoride toothpaste. Fluoride makes teeth more decay-resistant. It may also minimize the growth of bacteria. If using a special children's formula toothpaste makes it easier for your child to work up enthusiasm about brushing, fine. Gels, stripes, and sparkle formulas are big hits with kids. Just make sure that the toothpaste contains fluoride and is labeled with the seal of the American Dental Association.

My brother Bob, who is the proud father of three growing boys, also suggests that you may want to try a pump dispenser rather than a tube. A pump measures out the right amount, doesn't need to be recapped, and makes it easier to apply the toothpaste to the brush only—and not your bathroom walls!

Suppose your child hates the taste of toothpaste? Skip using toothpaste until your youngster finds it more palatable. It's the brushing action that gets teeth clean, not toothpaste. However, make sure that your child is getting an adequate amount of fluoride from other sources such as drinking water.

Brushing Permanent Teeth

When your child is about six years old, the tooth fairy will begin to make the first of many appearances. Baby teeth loosen and fall out. After a few weeks, permanent teeth begin to fill in the empty spaces. When you turn over the task of toothbrushing to your child, teach her the following steps.

- For proper brushing, show your child how to tilt the brush at a 45-degree angle against the gum line, with the head of the toothbrush next to his teeth. This places the bristles where plaque builds up.
- Make sure your child uses short, light, back-and-forth strokes to scrub the outer, inner, and chewing surfaces of each tooth.
- Be sure that your child applies just enough pressure to feel the tips of the bristles against the gums. Care should be taken not to squash the tips, since they do the work of brushing.

- Last, have your child lightly brush his tongue. This helps to remove bacteria from the mouth and sweetens breath. Be sure your child rinses well.
- Don't rush brushing. Your child's toothbrush can scrub only one or two teeth at a time. It takes three to five minutes to clean teeth thoroughly. Moving slowly ensures that your child's brush gets all surfaces of every tooth.

FACTS ON FLOSSING

For healthy teeth and gums your child also needs to floss to remove harmful plaque. The same plaque bacteria that damage adult gums are also present in children's mouths. Left unchecked, plaque buildup can lead to tooth decay and gum disease. Flossing does what a toothbrush can't. A toothbrush can't reach between teeth or under the gum line, areas where plaque hides and food particles get stuck.

When should flossing become a habit? As soon as all of your child's primary teeth have appeared, you can begin to do a daily flossing between any teeth that touch each other. Some baby teeth may have natural spaces between them; brushing alone is enough to loosen and sweep away any food particles.

Permanent teeth, of course, are larger. Because they take up more space, they touch each other, giving food particles and plaque snug hiding places. When your child's permanent teeth begin to come in, you need to be more diligent about thorough flossing. Include flossing as part of your child's toothbrushing routine at bedtime, and it will become a lifelong habit. Children are usually not ready to floss their own teeth until they are around ten years old. Even then, you should still supervise each flossing session.

To make flossing fun, you might want to choose one of the flavored flosses made for kids. Johnson and Johnson Dental Floss for Kids comes in a bright color and tastes just like bubble gum! For easy flossing, follow these simple steps.

FLOSSING HOW-TOS

1. Remove about eighteen inches of dental floss from the dispenser. Starting at one end, wrap most of it around the mid-

dle finger of the right hand if you are right-handed; the left hand if you are left-handed.
2. Wind the rest of the floss around the middle finger of the opposite hand. This finger will take up the soiled floss as the opposite finger unwinds each fresh section.
3. Next, hold about an inch of floss tightly between thumbs and forefingers. Tighten any slack.
4. Gently guide floss between teeth. At the gum line curve the floss into a **C** shape against one tooth. Gently slide floss between the gum and tooth.
5. With the floss held tightly against the tooth, use an up-and-down motion to slide just beneath the gum line and scrape the side of each tooth clean. Do not saw the floss back and forth.
6. Unwinding floss as you need to, continue to floss each tooth in this way. Don't overlook the back side of the last tooth in each row at the back of your child's mouth.
7. For thorough flossing, do your child's mouth in four sections. Floss the upper teeth on one side of her mouth, then the other. Repeat this pattern for the bottom teeth.
8. After flossing, have your child rinse her mouth to wash away loosened plaque.

After each of your child's first few flossing sessions her gums may bleed slightly and be sore. This is normal. As you break up plaque and remove bacteria, the gums will heal and bleeding will stop. If bleeding does not stop within the first five or six days of flossing, see your pediatric dentist. You may not be flossing properly. The key is to be thorough yet gentle.

YOUR CHILD'S FIRST DENTAL CHECKUPS

By taking your child to the dentist at an early age (between the ages of six and twelve months), you give your child a head start in developing good dental care habits—and you give your dentist a better shot at preventing future problems. For example, if your child loses a baby tooth prematurely, she may have to wear a space maintainer until the permanent tooth comes through the gums. This special appliance reserves a space for the incoming permanent tooth. Without a space maintainer the teeth beside the lost tooth may tilt toward the empty space. The result: the permanent teeth may come in crooked or crowded. Either condition may call for expensive, long-term treatment in the future.

When you consider the low cost of preventive services such as fluoride treatments and sealants compared to the higher expense of fillings, crowns, and other treatments, you'll see that it pays to get your child off to an early start. To make dental checkups go more smoothly, you may want to take your child to a pediatric dentist.

Pediatric dentists specialize in caring for the oral health of children from infancy through the teenage years. They are also qualified to give children with emotional, physical, or mental handicaps special care. And you'll be glad to know that the pediatric dentist works in tandem with pediatricians, other physicians, and other dental specialists. This team effort goes a long way to safeguard your child's overall health.

As for how often to visit the dentist, some children may need check-ups only every six months. However, because a child's dental needs depend on the individual, your pediatric dentist may suggest another timetable. Keep in mind that your child's need to go to the dentist depends on several factors: how clean he keeps his teeth, how well he eats, and whether or not he is getting enough fluoride. Your pediatric dentist will help you to keep track of your child's dental care needs.

What Happens During Your Child's First Visit

During your child's first dental visits, your pediatric dentist will go over the basics of dental hygiene. He or she will check your child's teeth and gums for decay and other problems. If your child already shows signs of damage, your dentist will give you ways to treat it at home.

X rays of your child's teeth may be taken to detect any hidden decay and to make sure that teeth and facial bones are developing properly.

Your child's teeth may be professionally cleaned, or a follow-up appointment for cleaning will be made if needed.

If your child has a habit of thumb sucking, the dentist can help to evaluate the problem. Your child's need for a balanced diet and for fluoride, a mineral that fights cavities, will also be discussed. And, of course, your pediatric dentist will show you how to clean your child's teeth on a daily basis, and teach you other home care skills that you need to keep your child's teeth and gums healthy and problem free.

Taking the Fear Out of Dental Visits

Small children sometimes find visits to the dentist scary. To make your child's trips more pleasant and relaxed for both of you, try to talk to him in an upbeat, positive way.

- Reassure your child that the dentist is a gentle, kind doctor who wants to keep his teeth and gums strong and healthy. If you yourself feel any anxiety about going to the dentist, try not to let it show. Your child is sensitive and will pick up on your "vibes."
- While you want your child to enjoy his visit to the dentist, don't offer bribes or rewards. He will assume that something unpleasant must be coming up.
- Actions speak louder than words. Be a good influence, and be diligent about your own brushing and flossing. And stick to your own dental appointments on a regular basis.

FLUORIDE: THE CAVITY FIGHTER

To fight cavities, your child needs fluoride, a mineral that combines with tooth enamel to strengthen teeth and make them more resistant to decay. Fluoride also works to repair some microscopic cavities, "healing" the tooth surface and making the enamel stronger than it was before. Some studies also show that fluoride may prevent or slow calcium loss from the bones. That would include the bone that supports the gums.

If the drinking water in your community is fluoridated, your baby may grow up to have 40 percent fewer cavities than children who don't drink fluoridated water. As your child drinks the water, the fluoride is absorbed into the developing teeth. *Note:* Infants who receive only breast milk or only commercial formula need fluoride supplements. Your dentist will be able to tell whether or not your child is getting enough fluoride to help her teeth grow strong and healthy. If her fluoride intake is inadequate, she can get it from other sources.

Other than optimally fluoridated drinking water, good sources include dietary supplements (drops for babies, chewable tablets and lozenges for children over one year old); fluoridated toothpaste (for children ages two and over); fluoride mouth rinses (for children ages six and over); at-home fluoride treatments (for children ages six and over); and professional fluoride treatments (for children ages three and over). Your pediatric dentist will let you know which, if any, of these choices your child needs.

Good news for parents of infants! One manufacturer of baby food, Beech-Nut, now offers Baby's First Spring Water, a sodium-free spring water with fluoride. It's meant to be used not only as baby's drinking water but also to mix with cereals, to dilute fruit juices, and to prepare infant formula. Ask your pediatrician or pediatric dentist for details, or call Beech-Nut at 1-800-523-6633.

Fluorosis

You've already read about how your child might develop fluorosis, a mottling of the teeth, if he gets more than his share of fluoride. This condition occurs only during the formation of your child's teeth, although you don't see it until the teeth erupt.

As you might have guessed, outbreaks of fluorosis are more prevalent in areas that have fluoridated drinking water. This is not because there is too much fluoride in the water, but because the child may also be swallowing too much toothpaste or getting too much fluoride from other sources. Of course, you want your child to get enough to prevent cavities. However, according to New York City dentist Jon C. Kellner, an overabundance of fluoride does *not* increase the antidecay effectiveness of fluoride in a significant way.

Fortunately, fluorosis does not affect the health of your child's teeth. But it may affect the appearance. To treat the discoloration of fluorosis, your dentist can remove a superficial layer of enamel. This is a slow process, taking about an hour and a half in the dentist's chair. But if your child is self-conscious about the way his teeth look, it's well worth the time and expense.

SEALANTS: HELP TO SEAL OUT DECAY

Children today have an extra advantage in the fight against cavities: sealants. A sealant is a clear or shaded plastic coating that is brushed on the chewing surfaces of the back teeth (premolars and molars). This area is particularly vulnerable to decay from plaque and acid buildup. The sealant works like a barrier to prevent attacks from the acids that form in plaque when sugar is eaten.

Why are the back teeth so susceptible to decay? As the back teeth develop, depressions and grooves (called pits and fissures) form in the chewing surfaces of the enamel. Because it's difficult for the bristles of a toothbrush to reach into these irregularities, it's nearly impossible to keep them clean. Plaque and bits of food get wedged in there to stay.

While fluoride works against decay on the smooth surfaces of the teeth, it can't do the job in the pits and fissures. Sealants cover these bumpy surfaces to seal them against the buildup of plaque and food. Since this treatment is most effective when applied to newly erupted teeth, children reap the greatest benefits from sealants. You can assure your child that applying sealants is a simple, painless procedure.

Although the sealant is invisible to the naked eye, you can rest assured that it's there, safeguarding your child's smile. In fact, it may be several years before your child needs a reapplication. Your pediatric dentist will do a routine check of sealants during regular office visits and will let you know if any need to be reapplied.

Having your child's teeth treated with sealants is another smart step in planning a well-rounded program of dental care. To be most effective, your child's plan should include the following: regular dental checkups; regular use of fluoride; daily brushing and flossing; sealants; and a healthy diet with a limited amount of sweets and sugar-rich foods.

If your child follows each one of these steps, he can beat the odds against cavities. Studies show that using fluoride and sealants together can wipe out tooth decay up to 90 percent. Now, that's quite a mouthful!

EATING RIGHT FOR HEALTHY TEETH

For strong, sound, cavity-resistant teeth, the right foods count. And it's not just what your child should not eat (sugars, sticky snacks) that matters, but also what he *should* eat. The nutrients your child takes in will help to keep teeth healthy.

A variety of foods should go into a balanced diet. Good sources of calcium, an important building block for strong teeth, are milk, cheese, and yogurt. Three glasses of milk a day provide all the calcium and phosphorus needed for developing teeth. And Cheddar cheese has a lot going for it. Studies show that it contains substances that neutralize the cavity-causing acids produced by bacteria in plaque!

Make sure your child also gets plenty of fruits and vegetables as well as bread and cereals and protein. And try not to give your child sugary foods. Honey, brown sugar, and syrups do as much harm to teeth as refined white sugar.

Smart Snacks

It may surprise you to know that even fresh fruits and vegetables can cause cavities! And so can the potato chips and pretzels that preteens love. Both sugary and starchy foods produce acids that attack tooth enamel and lead to decay. These acids go to work for twenty minutes, whether or not the food remains in the mouth. Also, it's not so much what your child eats as how often. The more your child snacks, the more often acid forms on her teeth.

Believe it or not, candy is no worse (and no better) than most munchies kids eat between meals. Even a sticky sweet such as a caramel dissolves and clears the mouth faster than a nutritious snack such as raisins or a potato chip or cracker. Cooked starches, such as breads, cereals, and crackers, stick to the teeth for hours until the enzyme *amylase* in the saliva breaks them down into sugars that can clear the mouth easily. Meanwhile, teeth are under attack from acids in the plaque.

Of course, you don't want your child to fill up on sweets or other empty calories. When your child gets the munchies, treat her to one of the following taste-pleasers: a hard-boiled egg; sugar-free peanut butter; chunks of Cheddar cheese; milk; plain yogurt; vegetable juice; slices of carrot and/or celery; pickles.

Brushing after snacking is ideal, although not always practical and possible. Your best bet is to keep your child's snacking moderate, no more than three or four items a day.

One last surprise: Chewing gum has always gotten a bad rap. However, studies show that chewing gum, whether sugared or sugar free, stimulates the flow of saliva, which helps to carry decay-causing bacteria from the teeth.

WHAT TO DO IF A TOOTH IS KNOCKED OUT

Your child scores a touchdown. Or takes a dive on his roller skates. Either way, he gets back on his feet with a missing tooth. Don't panic. If you act quickly, there's a good chance that your child's tooth can be saved. The following plan will help.

1. Retrieve the tooth. This may mean getting down on your hands and knees to do your hunting, but it's important to find the tooth.
2. Gently rinse the tooth in cold water if it's dirty. Do not scrub.
3. If the knocked-out tooth is a permanent one, try to insert it into its socket. To hold it in place have your child bite down on a clean cloth or piece of gauze. If the knocked-out tooth is a primary (baby) tooth, it should not be reimplanted. Nevertheless, the child and the tooth should be taken to a pediatric dentist.
4. If you cannot reposition the tooth, place it in a container of milk or cool water. (Milk gives the tooth a protective coating.) Or gently wrap the tooth in a clean wet cloth.

Keeping the tooth wet helps to preserve the vital tissue around the root. It also keeps the tooth from drying out. The tooth may look chalky compared to other teeth in your child's mouth if it loses moisture.
5. Take your child and the knocked-out tooth to your dentist pronto! If you get there within thirty minutes of the injury, the dentist may be able to replant the tooth and apply a splint. Call your dentist even if the accident occurs at night or over a weekend. If your dentist is not available, call a hospital emergency room.

Why is it so important to act within a half hour? After thirty minutes, the vital cells around the root of the tooth will begin to die quickly. Without those cells the tooth will be rejected by your child's body when the dentist tries to replant it.

Suppose it's not possible to get help within thirty minutes? To buy extra time, you may want to have on hand a product that will keep the vital cells of a tooth root alive for up to twenty-four hours. It's called Save-a-Tooth and consists of a nonbreakable screwtop jar containing a nontoxic sterile fluid formulated to nurture the cells around the tooth root. For information call 1-800-882-0505.

OTHER DENTAL INJURIES

If your child survives a spill without losing a tooth, you should still be on the lookout for damage. Even when a tooth is only chipped, you should take your child to the dentist as soon as possible. The tooth may need filing; prompt attention may also help to save the root.

To treat a broken tooth, rinse away any dirt or debris from the injured area with warm water. Place a cold compress over your child's face to reduce swelling over the broken tooth. And see your dentist immediately.

If the damage is minor, your dentist will smooth the rough edges of the broken tooth. For a more serious break, your dentist may medicate the tooth and cover it with a crown, metal band, or plastic material. Your dentist can rebuild fractured teeth to look as good as new and stabilize loose or displaced teeth.

Sometimes the damage resulting from a fall can go unnoticed. But it is possible that your youngster can still lose a tooth later on or develop bite problems due to hidden injuries beneath the gums. To play it safe, any injury to your child's mouth should be checked by your dentist.

Mouth Guards

Playing sports can also put your child's smile at risk. If you have young athletes in the family, have them fitted with a mouth guard. (This includes girls, too!) This appliance fits over the teeth and will help to prevent injury to your child's teeth, lips, cheeks, and tongue. A mouth guard also cushions blows to the head and neck that might result in concussions or jaw fractures.

You can find mouth guards at drug and sporting goods stores. One drawback: mass-produced mouth guards come in standard sizes and may fall short of a perfect fit. In that case you may want to have your child custom-fitted for a mouth guard by your dentist. Custom-fitted protectors earn high marks for the best fit, comfort, and quality. But as you might expect, they are more expensive. Whatever type of mouth guard you choose, it should be not only comfortable but also durable, resilient, tear-resistant, and thin enough to allow your child to breathe easily.

SMILE STRAIGHTENING: BASICS ON BRACES

When the smile that lights up your child's face shows off straight, healthy teeth, it certainly enhances his appearance. But there's more to having straight teeth than good looks—it can be very important for your child's good health.

Malocclusion ("bad bite") is the term dentists and orthodontists use to describe teeth that are out of alignment or that do not mesh properly when the jaws are closed; or it can be a combination of both conditions. A bad bite tends to run in families, but it can also be the result of missing teeth; sometimes the incoming teeth tip toward the empty space. And if your child sucks her thumb beyond the age of four or five, she can also develop a malocclusion.

Why is it so important to have straight teeth? Good question. Overlapping, crowded, crooked, or widely spaced teeth are harder to brush and floss, leaving teeth vulnerable to decay. When teeth are out of alignment it can cause excessive wear and tear, which may lead to *periodontic* problems (gum tissue abnormalities).

Some malocclusions can result in wearing of the tooth surface or lead to muscle tension and pain of temporomandibular joints (TMJ). These joints connect the lower jaw to the base of the skull. Popping and clicking jaws, headaches, and neck and facial pain are among the signs of TMJ disorders. When a child's teeth protrude, they may fracture more easily than straight teeth in the event of an accident.

Does this mean that if your child forgoes braces, he is sure to develop any of these problems? Not necessarily. Orthodontists can't make these predictions with 100 percent accuracy, but the risks may be greater if your child's problem goes uncorrected. Your pediatric dentist and pediatrician may advise you as to when to begin visits to the orthodontist. But you should also be on the lookout for any problems with your child's smile and can consult an orthodontist directly. The American Association of Orthodontics lists the following early warning signs that may signal the need for orthodontic care.

- Baby teeth falling out too early (before age five) or not on time (by age six)
- Difficulty in chewing or biting
- Mouth breathing (child has difficulty closing lips)
- Thumb sucking or tongue thrusting
- Crowded, misplaced, or blocked-out teeth
- Jaws that shift or make sounds
- Speech difficulty
- Biting into the cheek or into the roof of the mouth
- Protruding teeth
- Teeth that meet in an abnormal manner or don't meet at all
- Facial imbalance
- Jaws that protrude or recede
- Grinding or clenching of the teeth

Braces and Self-esteem

Crooked teeth or misaligned jaws can also make your child self-conscious about her appearance. This feeling may be particularly acute during the preteen years. If you notice that she tends to smile with her lips closed, or hides her mouth with her hand when she laughs or talks, she may be feeling ill at ease with her looks. Improving the health of your child's smile is also a boost to her self-confidence. When her teeth are straight and her jaws are properly aligned, she may feel more attractive and secure. Better self-esteem is one of the bonuses of proper orthodontic care.

Your Child's First Trip to the Orthodontist

The sooner a bite problem is detected and treated, the easier it is to prevent problems later on. Approximately one-third of your child's facial growth takes place between the ages of ten and twenty. And by the time he is twelve, your child should have all of his permanent teeth, except his third molars. Should your child have any problem with his bite, this is often a good time to begin treatment. However, your child may need the attention of an orthodontic specialist when she is as young as age two or three. (In some cases, pediatric dentists may treat some forms of malocclusions in young children.) As a rule, your child should make his first trip to the orthodontist no later than age seven.

Taking your child to an orthodontist at an early age does not necessarily result in early treatment. If the exam shows that all is well with your child, your orthodontist may simply recommend periodic followup visits. If your child does have a problem, the orthodontist will determine whether or not to treat the malocclusion now or to wait until a later age when there's been more growth.

Orthodontic care for young children is called *interceptive treatment*. Starting early allows the orthodontist to work with the natural growth of teeth and facial bones rather than against it. Young children are also less self-conscious about their looks, so it may be easier to get their cooperation in wearing any appliances. Another plus: early intervention can also speed up the completion of orthodontic treatment at a later age.

Basically, there are three stages of treatment, according to orthodontist Dr. Barton H. Tayer, clinical director of postgraduate orthodontics at Harvard University School of Dental Medicine.

Stage 1 is early treatment for children as young as two years of age (who may have such problems as cleft palate) up to age eleven. Criteria for treatment include skeletal disharmonies (the jaws are not growing harmoniously); cross bites (a front upper tooth that's behind a lower tooth when the jaws are closed), which can interfere with growth and development; severe crowding, which prevents your child from cleaning her teeth properly and can lead to gum problems; and severe protrusion. Your child's orthodontist can help him break abnormal habits at this time.

Stage 2 is treatment for youngsters from preadolescence into the teenage years and is performed to correct the typical kinds of malocclusion.

Stage 3 involves surgical correction. For this to be successful it may be necessary to wait until the jaws finish growing. If surgery is performed too early it may have to be repeated later on, as jaws and teeth are still developing.

Whatever stage of treatment your child needs, your orthodontist will best determine the goals and will choose the proper course for correcting her problem. In many cases the orthodontist will opt for either a removable or fixed appliance (braces) to get your child's smile on track.

Choosing an Orthodontist

Because the results of orthodontic treatment are permanent, you want to make sure that your child is in the expert hands of a specialist. There is also the expense to consider. Treatment can run from $2,000 to $4,000; you certainly want to get your money's worth!

Orthodontic specialists practice only orthodontics and have advanced training to manage the careful treatment of your child's teeth as well as guide the development of the face. Most orthodontists also make it easier for you to afford their fees by offering monthly payment plans.

To find an excellent orthodontist, ask your family dentist to refer you to an active member of the American Association of Orthodontists. You can also write to the association for a list of their members in your area. Write:

American Association of Orthodontists
401 North Lindbergh Boulevard
St. Louis, MO 63141

Update on Braces

"Tin Grin." "Metal Mouth." "Tinsel Teeth." These are some of the names you may have been teased with if you grew up with braces. But today braces are smaller, lighter, more comfortable, and less conspicuous than the "heavy metal" versions of the past. Wearing braces is so common now that it seems to have lost its social stigma. Instead, braces have taken on all the glamour of a status symbol with many youngsters.

How do braces work? They apply gentle pressure to move teeth into their proper positions. This steady force stimulates the body to make new tissue to support the new position of the teeth. Braces are sometimes called fixed appliances because they are attached directly to the teeth (as opposed to removable appliances), which gives the advantage of better control of tooth movement.

In some cases your child may have to wear a headgear while she sleeps. This is an elastic band that goes behind your child's neck or back of the head and fastens into an arch wire. The wire fits into tubes on bands attached to one or more teeth on each side of her upper jaw. The headgear helps to move teeth into normal positions or keeps certain teeth from moving at all.

How long does it take to fix a crooked smile? Length of treatment may vary from one to three years to achieve desired results. The average time frame is two years. The development of your child's face, how well she cooperates with treatment, and the seriousness of her problem all figure into determining how long she must wear her braces.

After discussing treatment and costs with you, your orthodontist will recommend the best braces for your child's smile. The following roundup of choices will give you a brief overview of the latest options available today.

Stainless Steel Braces

Made of stainless steel brackets and wire, standard stainless steel braces are made with a computerized machine and are considered to be the most efficient in terms of getting the best results. Because they are more flexible, they are more resistant to fracture than other materials used in making braces such as ceramics and plastics. Stainless steel braces also do a better job of rotating lower front teeth. They are also less expensive than other materials. Fees run from $2,800 to $4,000, depending on where you live and the length and complexity of treatment.

Minibraces

Minibraces are modern lightweight versions of the traditional stainless steel braces. Brackets are one-third the size and are bonded to the front of the teeth, doing away with the need for wearing elastic bands. But don't let the small size fool you. Minibraces are engineered to perform just as well as standard stainless steel braces. Because they are more delicate, minibraces are also more attractive than the standard model. The price range for minibraces is close to that of standard stainless steel braces.

Ceramic Braces

For the most natural look, there are ceramic braces, which are made of translucent or transparent material so that there's less contrast with teeth. Except for a stainless steel wire that runs across the teeth, ceramics are practically invisible.

Unlike stainless steel braces, ceramic braces are manufactured by firing in an oven. However, while they may be more pleasing to the eye than standard steel braces, they do not outdo them in performance. Both stainless steel and ceramics achieve the same results.

A few of the advantages of ceramic braces: They may be more comfortable than stainless steel. Because ceramic braces are clear, it is easier to spot any food particles. They are also stainproof, hypoallergenic, and do not conduct heat and cold.

On the downside, although ceramic braces are nine times harder than stainless steel, they are also less flexible and vulnerable to breakage. Treatment may take somewhat longer, and it costs more. Expect to pay another $300 to $500 over the cost of stainless steel braces.

Tip: Ceramic braces are available in colors such as hot pink, grape, and bright blue for trend-conscious kids who want to add spark to their smiles. But consider this: the ceramic bracket is attached directly to the tooth until the orthodontist removes the appliance. Your youngster may like neon pink today but become tired of it six months down the road. If your child wants to give her braces pizzazz, she can opt instead for colored elastics.

Elastics

Elastics are the rubber bands placed on braces to apply the pressure necessary to move teeth and jaws into their correct position. Without elastics, the process of smile straightening takes longer, so it is important that your child follow her orthodontist's instructions in wearing them.

Your child may complain that the elastics hurt her teeth. Explain to her that this happens because her teeth are moving, which will give her a beautiful new smile. Reassure her that the soreness will go away after a few days. And remind her that if she does not wear her elastics as instructed, the discomfort will last longer and that it will be harder to move her teeth.

The only time your child should remove her elastics is when she brushes her teeth, gums, and braces after meals. As soon as she's finished, the elastics should be reapplied, unless advised otherwise.

Caring for Braces

Once your child is fitted with braces, he and the orthodontist are partners. The orthodontist's efforts will straighten a crooked smile, but your child must take charge of keeping his teeth healthy and clean.

Certain crunchy and chewy foods such as peanut brittle, caramels, and bubble gum are off-limits. And if your child has a habit of chewing ice cubes, he needs to give it up. Using common sense, he can eat some crunchy foods such as apples as long as he takes small bites and doesn't bite down too hard. Most certainly your child needs to be more diligent about brushing his teeth.

Plaque and food particles trapped behind braces can make gums swollen, leave marks on the teeth, give your child bad breath, and, of course, cause cavities. Plaque buildup can also yellow the teeth. Brushing after every meal is ideal but not always possible. When your child can't brush, he should rinse his mouth well with water.

To get teeth and braces spotless, your child needs to do a thorough job of brushing and rinsing at least once a day, preferably at bedtime. It's up to you to see that your child follows through. To help, here a few pointers.

- For the best results, your child should use the toothpaste and toothbrush your orthodontist recommends.
- Be sure that your child brushes all surfaces of his teeth (fronts, backs, and tops). The orthodontist will also show your child how to clean under the wires of the braces.
- Remind your child not to skip brushing along the gum line. Plaque buildup here will make gums swollen and sore and more sensitive to brushing.
- Your child should also floss his teeth carefully. His cleaning routine may also include using a fluoride mouth rinse and/or water squirter to dislodge plaque.
- Once your child finishes brushing, he should rinse his mouth well with water.
- After rinsing, your child should check his teeth, gums, and braces for any traces of plaque. Since he has to take a close look, make sure your bathroom mirror is well lighted.

Bear in mind that your child needs to keep up with regular dental checkups as well as her routine visits to the orthodontist. If you notice that your child's elastic bands break frequently, or that a wire or band loosens, or a hook breaks off her braces, call your orthodontist at once. Correcting these mishaps as soon as possible is important to keeping on track with your child's progress.

Removable Appliances

Not every bite problem is corrected with fixed braces. In some cases the orthodontist will recommend a removable appliance, a device made of plastic and wire. Unlike fixed appliances (braces) that attach directly to the teeth to apply gentle pressure, removable appliances work in different ways, depending on the type of appliance used.

Sometimes removable appliances can be used as an alternative to braces if the bite problem is minor. In this case, your child can wear a special tooth-moving appliance, a device that fits over the teeth. Like braces, it puts pressure on teeth until they arrive at the proper position. Sometimes a tooth-moving appliance is used to begin the smile-straightening process before a child is ready for braces. A few advantages: the appliance can be popped out for eating and for cleaning.

The retainer is the most commonly used removable appliance. Once your child's braces are removed, the retainer holds teeth in their corrected position. Your child may need to wear one for a year or more on a full-time basis, or only part time—for example, during sleep—for several months.

If your child clenches his jaws or grinds his teeth he may need a bite plane. This device separates teeth in the back of the mouth along the upper and lower jaw. It keeps the teeth from meeting when jaws are closed. Another bad-habit buster is the Thumb Guard. As you may have guessed, it helps to put a stop to thumb sucking. But Dr. Barton H. Tayer advises that this device be used only if thumb sucking is a problem and only if your child wants to give it up. Splints help to relieve the clicking, popping, or pain around the ear in the temporomandibular joints (TMJ) by relaxing the jaw muscles and making teeth more comfortable.

Keep in mind that in order to achieve the best results, your child has to wear (not remove) her removable appliance. Otherwise jaws, teeth, and muscles can revert to their original positions.

To build your child's confidence, remind her that she needs to take a little time to get used to her appliance. Your child might lisp at first or have another speech impediment. Eating can feel unnatural. She may also feel that she has more saliva in her mouth. With a little encouragement from you, your child will eventually get used to wearing her appliance. And then it will become easier for her to stick with her program—and gain a gorgeous grin!

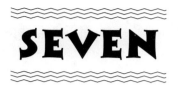

SEVEN

Eyes Right! Eye Care and Eye Wear for Kids

YOUR CHILD'S EYESIGHT is precious. You want your child to see the world clearly, with eyes that are bright and shining with good health.

Your child needs good vision to become familiar with the faces of loved ones, to become acquainted with shapes, colors, and textures, to engage in play, to read, to maneuver her way through the world, to act independently—in short, to map out her daily life with ease and confidence.

This chapter will give you the guidelines you need to take care of your child's eyes. You'll learn when to begin eye checkups for your child, how to tell whether your child may be having problems with his vision, the basics of eye safety and first aid for eye care emergencies.

Does your child need glasses? This chapter will help you to choose flattering frames that fit and that can take the everyday wear and tear inflicted by active kids. You will also find the answers to many questions parents have about good vision care: "What is 'lazy eye,' and can it be cured?" "Is watching TV bad for my child's eyes?" "My child hates wearing glasses—how can I help?" "Are contact lenses safe for kids?"

HERE'S LOOKING AT YOU, KID!

Take a closer look at the essentials of eye care today, and you will be better equipped to teach your child how to protect his vision as he grows up.

THE VIEW FROM YOUR BABY'S WORLD

How well does a newborn see? Until recently many experts believed that what infants saw was nothing more than a dim gray blur. Today we know that a baby is born with all of the biological structures needed for sight.

As light passes through the *cornea* (the outermost surface of the eye), the flexible, transparent tissue of the *lens* focuses it onto the *retina*, the thin, light-sensitive membrane at the back of the eyeball. In response to this light, nerve cells on the retina will send signals along the optic nerve. In this way, information about the object your baby views is carried to the brain.

While the mechanisms for sight are the same in an infant's eye as they are in an adult's, the world through the eyes of a newborn looks somewhat different than it appears to you and me. For example, objects more than eight to fifteen inches away from a baby's nose may look blurry. (Many experts believe that a baby learns to recognize his mother's face first because she is no farther than eight inches away when cradling her baby for a feeding. This may explain why babies prefer to look at closer objects.)

Distance vision is fuzzy because the lens of a newborn lacks the ability to change its shape as the baby's eye focuses on faraway objects. (The lens thickens to focus on near objects and needs to become thinner in order to focus on objects at a distance.) And since the distance between the cornea and the retina of a newborn's eye is shorter than it is in an adult's eye, the retinal image will be smaller. As a result, it won't be easy for your infant to tell exactly how big the object is.

Your infant also lacks full control of the muscles around her eyes. This may make it hard for her to align both eyes on the same thing. One of baby's eyes may even wander out of focus. But by two months of age your baby learns to use both eyes together, and this random movement should stop. (If not, your baby may have a vision problem called *strabismus*. For more information, see pages 150–51.)

Eyes Right!

Once your baby is two to three months old, she will fix her gaze on faces and close objects. You will also see that she follows moving objects with her eyes. At four months of age your baby will not only be able to make out the shapes and sizes of close objects, but will reach out to touch and grasp what she sees. By the time your baby is six months old, her vision should allow her to identify and distinguish between objects.

Does your newborn see colors? Not all the color receptors in the retina are working efficiently. But studies show that before your infant is three months old, he can probably see reds and greens, and possibly blues. Once he is four months old, he should be able to recognize colors in the same hue groupings as adults.

Eye-pleasers for Babies

What does your baby like to look at? Research shows that simple geometric patterns and high-contrast designs catch an infant's eye, hence the vogue for chic black-and-white toys and nursery furnishings for newborns. Gazing at faces is especially appealing, and so is looking into mirrorlike surfaces (including your eyes). Sources of light are also attractive to infants.

The objects that fascinate your baby can also stimulate his vision. Here are a few attention-getting objects and tips on how to use them.

- Toys, stuffed animals, and mobiles in simple black-and-white geometric patterns have lots of eye appeal for newborns.
- Playthings in cheerful primary colors such as clear red, bright blue, and sunny yellow can be introduced by the time your infant is a few months old.
- Objects that move, such as mobiles and rattles, delight baby's eye. So do visual displays in bold graphic patterns and shapes.
- A nonbreakable mirror is a must. By six months of age, babies love to look at themselves!

When decorating baby's room, don't go overboard with lots of black and white or a riot of primary colors. This sensory overload acts like visual noise and can be less than soothing for your infant. Her eyes need a break from "sight-seeing," and keeping the nursery calm and restful helps.

Your infant is also more intrigued with small objects, such as a rattle, than she is with a big wall hanging across the room. A few small items in baby-pleasing colors are all the visual stimulation she needs.

To sum up, you don't need to invest in lots of visually correct amusements for your baby. The world around her will provide plenty of visual delights and lessons to promote normal growth and development.

FOCUS ON EYE CHECKUPS

Just as your child needs routine trips to his dentist and pediatrician, he also needs regular eye exams. Eye checkups will help to keep his vision clear and sharp (and to correct it if it is not) and to make sure that his eyes are healthy. The American Academy of Ophthalmology and the American Optometric Association both recommend early evaluation of an infant's eyes.

A newborn's eyes should be examined for general eye health by a pediatrician or family physician. Infants at high risk should be examined by an ophthalmologist (a medical doctor who has completed residency in diagnosing and treating eye disorders) or an optometrist (a doctor of optometry) who specializes in the examination, diagnosis, and treatment of infants' and children's eye and vision problems. You should also know that all premature children are at a greater risk than normal children for developing such problems as *myopia* (nearsightedness), *strabismus* (misaligned or crossed eyes), and *astigmatism* (an irregularity of the cornea that results in blurred vision). Eye checkups for high-risk children should be routine throughout childhood.

By the time your baby is six months old, she should be screened for ocular health by an ophthalmologist or optometrist. (Also, your pediatrician should make an eye screening a routine part of every checkup.) Along with testing your little one's vision, an exam by a pediatric eye specialist also checks for signs of eye disease, proper alignment of your child's eyes, and whether or not both eyes are working together. If your baby's eyes seem to be developing normally, she won't need more formal vision testing until she is three or four years old.

Your baby's visual cells develop quickly between the ages of one and two years. If your toddler's vision is normal, by the time she has her second birthday, she can probably see at the 20/40 level. This measurement of visual activity (how clearly you distinguish details and shapes), based on the standard E-vision chart test, means that if your child can just see at a distance of twenty feet an object that a mature eye can see clearly at forty feet, she has 20/40 vision.

When your child is about three and a half years old, he should be tested for eye health and vision development by a ophthalmologist, optometrist, pediatrician, or family physician. (Between the ages of three and five, your child's vision develops to the 20/20 level.) It becomes easier to measure vision at this age because your child has better verbal skills and can describe what he sees. He can also follow any directions given to perform visual tasks, such as tracking moving objects. This makes test results more accurate. If testing shows that your child's visual range hasn't reached the expected level, your pediatrician will refer you to an optometrist or ophthalmologist.

At age five your child should have a preschool vision and motility (eye movement) evaluation. It's important to have your child examined in the preschool years, because most serious ocular conditions detected by routine screening can be found—and treated—then. Beyond age five, your child's eyesight should be examined routinely at in-school vision screenings or by a doctor if symptoms of eye problems show up. It is especially important to have your child's eyes checked if there is a history of vision problems in your family or among your relatives.

Between the ages of three and five, a child without impaired vision should be able to see at the 20/20 level, the same as adults. The development of your child's visual and visual-motor systems are usually completed by the age of eight or nine. Once these systems are fully developed, it's much more difficult to reverse or correct many eye and vision problems. You can understand why it is so critical to have any problems detected and treated at an early age.

Ideally, all children from birth to age three should be examined by a pediatric ophthalmologist or optometrist. According to pediatric ophthalmologist John Flynn, M.D., of Bascomb Palmer Eye Institute, University of Miami Medical School, this is not always practical. Dr. Flynn advises that if there are no signs of vision problems, your child's pediatrician can perform routine eye checkups. However, if there is any suspicion that anything is wrong, your child should be seen by an ophthalmologist or optometrist.

In-school Vision Screening

Once your child starts school, make regular eye exams part of your child's back-to-school routine. The school system in your community should provide regular vision screening programs.

These school checkups are performed by professional screeners, school nurses, and/or trained lay volunteers. During a school screening your child is asked to read an eye chart or perform other screening tests and answer questions that may reveal he has a vision problem. School screenings may detect the following: reduced vision in one eye due to amblyopia ("lazy eye"); uncorrected refractive errors such as nearsightedness and farsightedness; misalignment or crossing of the eyes (strabismus); or other eye defects.

Keep in mind that while eye checkups given at schools can find some vision problems such as nearsightedness, they are not a substitute for thorough eye exams conducted by a doctor. For example, most in-school screenings don't test for color blindness and don't include an exam of general eye health. And they can't identify the causes of vision problems. But should a vision problem be detected, a quality screening program will point you in the right direction for treatment.

SIGNS OF VISION PROBLEMS: WHEN TO CALL THE DOCTOR

Children don't always complain about having blurred or double vision or other eye problems. My friend Kathleen tells me that as a child she thought it was perfectly normal that the leaves she heard rustling in the trees were a soft haze of pale green. And then, to her delight, her first pair of glasses revealed that each leaf was separate and had a distinctive shape, with veins and edges that looked as if they'd been artfully cut with scissors. She never knew what she'd been missing!

How can you tell whether or not your school-age child is having trouble with her eyesight? The way she behaves may indicate the presence of a vision problem. The American Optometric Association recommends that you be on the alert for the following clues:

- Rubbing eyes excessively
- Blinking more than normal
- Constant squinting
- Difficulty in performing simple tasks such as tying shoelaces or buttoning clothing
- Short attention span
- Complaining of dizziness, headache, or nausea after reading, doing homework, or other close-up work
- Sitting too close to the television set
- Tripping while going up steps
- Shunning sports activities
- Avoiding reading, writing, drawing, and other forms of close work

If your child shows any of the above signs, she may have an eye or vision problem—a trip to the pediatrician or eye doctor is in order. Other warning signs of possible eye problems are inflamed or watery eyes; eyelids that are red, swollen, or encrusted; recurring infections of eyelids; sensitivity to light; pupils of unequal size; drooping eyelids; and holding the head in an abnormal or twisted position.

You should also have your child's eyes examined if he complains of double or blurry vision or seems to have difficulty with color vision. Any eye injury, no matter how minor, needs medical attention. And if your child's eyes appear to be crossed or misaligned, he should definitely see an eye doctor. The sooner an eye problem is diagnosed, the better the odds are for correction.

COMMON VISION PROBLEMS AND HOW THEY ARE CORRECTED

Your child's eye checkup may reveal that she has faulty eyesight. The good news is that many vision problems are treatable. Should your child need corrective glasses, surgery, or other treatment, your eye doctor will give you the detailed information you need regarding your child's condition and the proper treatment.

In the meantime, it helps to know what some of the common vision problems are and what can be done to correct them.

AMBLYOPIA

Four-year-old Kathryn seems to have normal eyesight. She can dress herself, loves to play games, and can read numbers and letters. But if you cover her left eye, her world becomes a blur. Kathryn has amblyopia in her right eye.

Sometimes called "lazy eye," amblyopia is the term used to describe poor vision in an eye that did not develop normal sight during early childhood. The brain recognizes the image from the eye with good eyesight and "shuts off" the image from the weaker eye. If the problem is treated during infancy or early childhood, it *can* usually be fully corrected.

During early childhood, your child's vision continues to develop if she uses her eyes properly. She needs to aim both eyes at the same target to allow the visual part of her brain to fuse the two pictures into a single three-dimensional image. However, if she has poor vision in one eye, and relies solely on her good eye, normal binocular (two-eyed) vision can't develop properly and may actually decrease.

By the time your child is eight or nine years old her visual development is complete. If your child's amblyopia is not treated early, the "lazy" eye may develop a serious and irreversible visual defect. Your child may experience loss of depth perception. Should the good eye become injured or diseased, your child may have to face a lifetime of poor and uncorrectable vision. Because your child needs equal vision in both eyes in order to see well, early diagnosis and proper treatment are musts!

Causes of Amblyopia

Any condition that interferes with visual development and affects normal use of the eye can result in amblyopia. The three major causes are: strabismus (misaligned eyes); unequal focus (refractive errors such as nearsightedness that are more pronounced in one eye); cloudiness in the normally clear lens of the eye.

About half the children who have strabismus will develop amblyopia (see pages 150–51 for more on strabismus). One eye may turn in or out, up or down. If the same eye continually turns, amblyopia may result in that eye.

A refractive error is much harder to detect. If one of your child's eyes is out of focus because it is more nearsighted, farsighted, or astigmatic than the other, this eye "turns off," becoming lazy. Even though this eye has poor vision, the eye can look normal. (This was the case with Kathryn.)

This makes amblyopia difficult to detect and calls for thorough measurement of your child's vision by a pediatrician or eye doctor (ophthalmologist or optometrist). If amblyopia or misaligned eyes run in your family, have your child checked before the age of three.

Cloudiness of the lens is another cause of amblyopia. Any condition that keeps light from being clearly focused inside your child's eye can lead to amblyopia. If your pediatrician has any difficulty measuring vision or detects any sign of amblyopia or a related condition, your child will be referred to an ophthalmologist or optometrist.

Will correcting the cause of amblyopia cure it? Unfortunately, not always. Your eye doctor can correct blurred vision with glasses, remove a cataract, or straighten misaligned eyes, but the amblyopia must be treated separately.

Treating Amblyopia

If tests show that your child does have poor vision in one eye, does that mean that he has amblyopia? Not necessarily. Sometimes faulty vision can improve with glasses. But your ophthalmologist or optometrist will also examine the inner eye for other causes of decreased vision such as cataracts, inflammation, tumors (which are rare), or other disorders.

To treat amblyopia, your eye doctor may prescribe glasses to correct errors or imbalances in focusing. If this does not work, then your child has to wear a patch or covering over his good eye for a while. Wearing a patch forces your child to use his lazy eye. In not being able to favor his good eye, he will exercise the "lazy" eye so that it can develop good vision. Along with use of the patch, your child may need to perform various eye exercises, called vision therapy, to help develop better use of the two eyes together. In order for the patch treatment to succeed, your child may have to wear it for weeks or months. A followup of part-time patching is usually necessary to maintain restored vision.

This may be tough for you to enforce. It's especially frustrating for a toddler or preschooler to have to cope with blurry or hazy vision. To step up a young child's motivation, pediatric ophthalmologist Susan Day, M.D., suggests that you offer your child small but special rewards. For example, make a calendar with a colorful sticker or shiny star for each day she wears her patch. Or link wearing the patch with a positive activity. If your child wants to play Nintendo, she can only do so if she wears the patch during the game.

Your child has the best chances of improving his vision if the amblyopia is detected and treated early. Amblyopia can begin at birth or develop later—for example, around three years of age. By the age of six it is more difficult to reverse the condition. However, if loss of vision is due to misaligned eyes or unequal refractive errors (nearsightedness, farsightedness, astigmatism), it may be treated successfully at a much older age than the lazy eye that results from opacities in the eye. According to Dr. Susan Day, it is still worth pursuing treatment up to the age of twelve.

NEARSIGHTEDNESS

When six-year-old Nancy first sees her mother's face as she comes down the stairs it is a smudge; then gradually her mother's face comes into focus as she gets closer to her. Nancy is nearsighted.

Nearsightedness or *myopia* is the inability to see objects at a distance clearly. It is often inherited and is a common vision problem among young children. Children like Nancy see close objects better than those that are faraway. When light rays enter the eye, they focus in front of the retina. As a result, it is difficult to see faraway objects.

What causes nearsightedness? In most cases, an eyeball that's longer than average. This makes it difficult for the lens to focus on objects at a distance. Sometimes nearsightedness is caused by a change in the shape of the cornea or lens.

Luckily, nearsightedness is easy to treat. Wearing corrective lenses—either prescription eyeglasses or contact lenses—will bring your child's world into focus. During childhood, when your child shoots up quickly, it may be necessary to replace his glasses or lenses as often as every six months to keep up with his rapid rate of growth. Unfortunately, nearsightedness may get worse very quickly for several years, particularly during adolescence. This is not unusual. The good news is that more frequently myopia develops in low or moderate degree and stabilizes.

FARSIGHTEDNESS

Eight-year-old Sam often gets mild headaches after a reading binge. He has a severe case of *hyperopia*, or farsightedness. Sam can see faraway objects better than those close up, such as type on a page, because light rays entering the eye focus *behind* the retina. This is due to the eyeball's being shorter than average. As a result, the lens has difficulty in focusing on nearby objects.

It is normal for most children to be farsighted to some degree; but just as they can see objects clearly at a distance, they can also focus on close objects. As children develop, the eyeball elongates and the farsightedness decreases.

In most cases, children do not need glasses or contact lenses to correct this condition. However, children like Sam who complain of eye discomfort or headaches after reading or close work may have a more serious case and need to see an ophthalmologist or optometrist at once. Your child's farsightedness should also be corrected if the problem is associated with misaligned eyes. Corrective glasses or contact lenses will bring blurry close-up objects into focus.

ASTIGMATISM

Seen without eyeglasses, the world is a soft blur to five-year-old Jane. She has astigmatism. Objects that are at a distance or close up look blurry or wavy because light rays entering the eye scatter and focus at different places.

Light can't focus at a single point because the front surface of the eye, the cornea, is not perfectly round, and/or the curvature of the lens is uneven. Astigmatism often occurs with nearsightedness or farsightedness. For most children with astigmatism, wearing corrective glasses is the solution.

When and if your child is ready to wear contact lenses, she may be a candidate for *toric* contact lenses, special lenses designed to correct astigmatism, which come in soft and rigid materials. (For more information on contact lenses, see pages 159–65.)

STRABISMUS

You may have noticed that your newborn's eyes tend to cross in or out. In most cases, the muscles controlling eye movement aren't strong enough yet to work together. This is normal, but within a few weeks this random wandering should stop. If it does not, your child may have *strabismus*, a visual defect caused by eyes that are misaligned because of an imbalance in the muscles that control eye movement.

Symptoms of Strabismus

While one eye looks straight ahead, the other eye turns inward, outward, upward, or downward. Sometimes this misalignment may come and go. Or at times the straight eye may turn and the turned eye may straighten. While eye care experts don't fully understand the exact cause of this misalignment, they surmise that the muscles controlling the movement of the turned eye may be weaker than those of the straight eye.

If your child literally can't see straight, the brain accommodates this fault by blocking out the image from the turned eye. This causes amblyopia and loss of normal depth perception. (When adults develop strabismus they may have double vision; in an adult the brain can't "turn off" the image from the turned eye as easily.)

Because the brain controls eye movement, children with disorders that affect the brain (such as cerebral palsy, Down's syndrome, hydrocephalus, and brain tumors) often develop strabismus. Other causes of strabismus are a cataract, excessive farsightedness, or eye injury that affects your child's vision.

The most noticeable symptom of strabismus is a turned eye, though sometimes the turn is not very obvious. Kids are so adaptable that you may not notice any changes in the way they use their eyes. Other signs include squinting one eye in bright sunshine or tilting the head in a certain direction in order to use the eyes together. Of course, the best way to tell whether or not your child has true strabismus is to take him to the pediatrician or pediatric ophthalmologist or optometrist.

Treating Strabismus

Treatment for strabismus may include surgery to adjust the position of the eye muscles. Other eye-straightening measures include corrective eyeglasses, eye drops, special ointment, or prisms (a special type of lens). For some children, eye exercises may help them focus their eyes.

While surgery straightens the eyes, it does not take the place of treatment for amblyopia. Your child may still need to wear glasses or prisms or have amblyopia therapy.

COLOR BLINDNESS

Roses are red and the grass is green, but to those born with abnormal color vision the hues of these natural wonders can appear almost alike or, in rare cases, as shades of gray. The term "color-blind" is not entirely accurate, but it is commonly used to describe defective perception of color.

Eight percent of boys and fewer than one percent of girls have faulty color vision at birth. This inability to recognize colors ranges from slight to total loss of color vision. In many cases it is the red and green areas of the color spectrum that cannot be distinguished. You may not even notice that your child has defective color vision unless he makes glaring mistakes in identifying colors past the stage when he should know his colors.

What causes color blindness? A simplified explanation of how the eye perceives color will help you to understand this condition. The retina of the eye contains elements for sight called *rods* and *cones*. The rods function when lighting is dim and allow you to see at night. The cones function in daylight and allow you to see colors. The three types of cone pigments—blue, green, and red—work in harmony to allow you to see a marvelous spectrum of color.

Heredity controls the formation of each cone pigment. If your child inherits an abnormal gene, it may slightly change a particular pigment or do away with it completely. As a result your child could have trouble identifying certain colors such as reds and greens.

While defective color vision is often hereditary, there may be other causes. Retinal or optic nerve disease can trigger a change in color vision. If you think your child is "blind" to certain colors, consult your eye doctor, who will test your child's color sense.

The best time to have a color vision deficiency checked is before your child begins school. During the primary grades, many of the learning materials used are color coded. If your child cannot cope and teachers are not aware of his problem, he may be considered a slow learner.

Although hereditary defective color vision cannot be cured, you can help your child compensate for what he doesn't see. The following tips for parents and teachers are recommended by the American Optometric Association.

- Label each of your child's crayons, markers, and colored pencils with its color. This may help him to recognize colors by their names rather than by their appearance.
- To help your child put together a color-coordinated outfit by himself, label each article of clothing with the name of its color. If your child is not old enough to read, use a special symbol in place of the word.
- Name that color! Always refer to the objects you point out to your child by color. It is possible for many color-blind children to learn their colors, although the hue they see may be less intense or otherwise different from what children with normal color vision see.

- To help your child learn to read the colors on a traffic light, teach him the order of the lights that signal "Stop," "Wait," and "Walk." Show him how to identify which light is working by illumination rather than by its color.

A little praise from you also goes a long way toward helping your child to overcome his color vision deficiency. Compliment your child's efforts, and do not make him feel inadequate about his color vision problems. It may hearten you to know that many famous painters have been color-blind and have enriched the world by turning their abnormal sense of colors into breathtaking works of art!

GETTING INTO GLASSES

How well I remember my first pair of glasses! They were pale pink and had a habit of sliding down my nose. Since I was four years old at the time, my parents assumed most of the responsibility for wiping off the fingerprints and peanut butter smears that invariably smudged the lenses. And more than once my glasses had to be replaced when I accidentally sat on them!

Getting the right glasses for your child's eyes begins with a trip to the ophthalmologist or optometrist for a complete eye exam. (An *ophthalmologist* is a medical doctor—M.D.—who can examine eyes, prescribe drugs, measure eyes for glasses and contact lenses, and perform eye surgery. An *optometrist* is a doctor of optometry—O.D.—who can examine eyes, prescribe glasses, and fit contact lenses. While in some states optometrists treat certain diseases with drugs, they are not medical doctors and cannot perform surgery.)

If your child needs glasses, your eye doctor will write a prescription for the proper lenses. You may be able to obtain the glasses from the examining doctor or you can take the prescription to an optical shop where technicians will follow the prescription to grind or manufacture the correct lenses.

To make sure your child's prescription is accurate, always have it double-checked. The doctor's office will check the glasses before they are dispensed or you can have the glasses examined at the optical shop where they were purchased (the service is usually free) or take them elsewhere for a minimal fee (five dollars or less). Should your child's prescription be "off," take the glasses back to the shop where you purchased them. The problem will be corrected at no charge.

Frames That Fit

Six-year-old Annie's glasses keep sliding down her nose. Eight-year-old Josh, who loves the thrills and spills of soccer, has trashed three pairs of glasses in a year. And three-year-old Rachel often yanks her glasses off with one hand, stretching the temple out of shape.

All of these problems can be solved if the frames of your child's glasses are a good fit and if they are designed to withstand the kind of wear and tear that only active kids can inflict! If your child's frames stay put, it helps your child to adjust to the whole idea of wearing glasses. Your optician will work with you and your child in selecting the best frames for your child. Meanwhile, consider the following:

- For frames that fit, consider frames with an adjustable "unifit" bridge made of soft silicone. This allows each side of the bridge to adjust independently to fit the contours of your

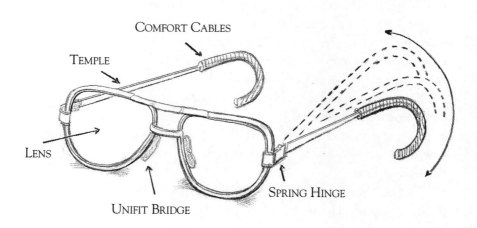

child's nose. It also prevents the bridge from pressing or pinching the nose.
- Other excellent options for good fit: rolled or flared nose pads, or silicone pads with a nonskid surface. You can also get rocking horse nose pads and arms drilled into the nose bridge. A bridge that fits well will distribute the weight of the frames evenly so that glasses stay straight and rest evenly on the face.
- Spring hinges on the side bars (temples) make the hinge area more flexible, allowing the temples to bend out as well as in. This feature compensates for a young child's tendency to pull her glasses away from her head with one hand. Since frames can maintain their shape, they won't slip down your child's nose.
- Comfort cables (cable temples) help to keep glasses on without pressing on the sides of the head. Flexible metal ear tips covered by rubber tubing curl comfortably around the ears.
- Kidproof frames should be made of materials that are sturdy, impact-resistant, thin, and lightweight. Carbon fiber graphite frames fit the bill. So do polymer frames.
- Another good choice: bendable, flexible frames made with a memory-encoded titanium alloy called Flexon. Your child could bend the bridge in half or twist the frames, and they would still go back to their original shape.

Flattering Frames

Eye-catching frames that are fun to wear will also step up your child's motivation to wear glasses. I speak from experience. As a young child, wearing frames in pretty colors and exotic shapes such as glamorous cat's eyes helped me to shrug off the taunts and teasing. My favorite pair of glasses came in a wild leopard print! They did not exactly complement my pressed and starched primary-color school clothes, but my mother indulged me. She knew that if I liked my glasses, I'd be more enthusiastic about wearing them.

If your child is concerned with the way he looks in glasses, you will want to make sure you pick a shape that flatters his face shape and shows off his features. For example, small faces would be overpowered by bold, chunky shapes. Thin, delicate frames are best. On the other hand, big, wide frames flatter long faces. In some cases, a frame shape that is the opposite of your child's facial contours will balance his features for the most attractive effect. On the following page, you will find some helpful guidelines for choosing frames.

Don't be surprised if your child passes up frames that flatter his face for another shape and style. He might look terrific in rectangles but prefer the round, preppie frames that are all the rage with his friends. In that case, don't try to dissuade him. What matters is that he wants to wear the glasses and will feel that he's in control if you go along with his choice.

Helping Your Child Adjust to Wearing Glasses

Not all children who need glasses have to wear them full time. Your child may need glasses only for reading and close work. Your eye doctor will let you know what your child's needs are and whether or not she has to wear them for certain activities.

Getting an infant or toddler to keep her glasses on may be tricky. After you slip them on, try to distract her. If she takes them off, gently replace them. And if this doesn't work, relax. Put the glasses away and give it another try later on. Trying to force a baby or toddler to wear glasses will get you nowhere. If your child persists in removing her glasses, they may not fit properly. The prescription may also need to be rechecked. (Perhaps the prescription is too strong, and your child is fussy because she can't see properly.) If getting your little one's cooperation continues to be a no-win situation, consult your eye doctor.

Coping with Teasing: Glasses and Your Child's Self-image

"Four Eyes!" "Mr. Peepers!" "Wimp!" Like many children who wear glasses, seven-year-old David gets his share of schoolyard teasing. Although the jokes are often meant in fun, they do take their toll on David's self-esteem.

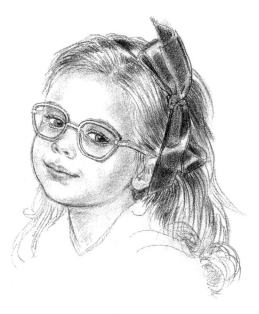

Many children have round faces. The planes and angles of rectangular or geometric frames will help to flatter this face shape.

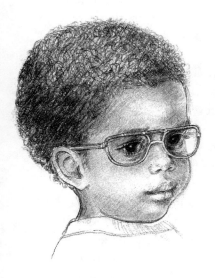

Aviators balance the narrow chin of a heart-shaped face.

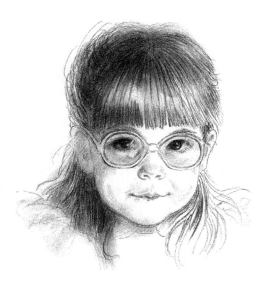

Frames in oval or round styles soften the lines of a square face.

Depending on your child's age and whether or not "specs" are a status symbol among his friends, wearing glasses can be at odds with his self-image. To help your child feel better about wearing glasses, be sensitive to his feelings. It helps if you can remember the childhood ribbings you got from your own schoolmates. Letting your child know how you coped can be reassuring.

Explain that sometimes children can be thoughtless and uncomfortable about others who are different from them. If your child understands that kids who taunt and tease do so out of insecurity, it may be easier for him to shrug off name-calling. And once his friends realize they can't unnerve your child with their jokes, the teasing may stop altogether.

Stress that wearing glasses is important. That your child will learn faster, perform better, and have more fun playing because it will be easier for him to see. Make it clear that his safety and well-being are more important than being teased.

Does your child have any four-eyed heroes? Favorite sports personalities, movie stars, or television celebrities who don specs may spark more interest in wearing glasses.

Look into glasses that are fun to wear and that are specifically designed for children. For example, frames with decals of sprightly Walt Disney characters are available for youngsters ages three to ten.

If you have glasses, make sure you wear them according to your doctor's orders. All the coping strategies in the world won't work if your child sees that you seem reluctant to wear your own glasses. Be a good example!

TLC for Glasses

Glasses may be fun to wear, but they're not toys! Teach your child to handle her glasses with care. These simple steps will help.

- Show your youngster how to use both hands to gently slip her glasses off her face. Pulling them off with one hand puts too much wear and tear on the temple.
- If your child needs to put her glasses down for a while, show her these three options: 1. Fold the sidepieces in and place

glasses lens side up. 2. Extend the sidepieces and place glasses right side up. 3. Extend the sides and place glasses with the brow bar down.
- For scratchproof cleaning, have your youngster place her glasses under tepid or cool running water. Liquid soap and a soft cloth may also be used if lenses are especially grimy.
- Dry off glasses with a clean, soft cloth. Remind your child not to use paper towels or tissue—they have tiny fibers that can scratch the lenses.
- Teach your youngster to keep her glasses in a safe place when she's not wearing them. A padded case will protect against scratching and breakage. Some cases come with a handy key chain hook that snaps onto a belt or backpack, great for on-the-go kids.

A LOOK AT CONTACT LENSES

Are contact lenses safe for children? That depends on many factors. Infants and young children who have surgery for congenital cataracts are fitted with a very powerful, pediatric contact lens. (Thick glasses can be used but cause magnification and distortion.) Contact lenses are also prescribed for children to treat birth injuries and to correct visual defects such as crossed eyes, amblyopia, and nearsightedness. However, when contact lenses are used as an alternative to glasses, many children aren't ready to take care of them until the preteen years.

Whether or not your child is ready to wear contact lenses depends less on his age and more on his desire to wear them and his ability to take care of them. Switching to contacts should be *his* idea, not only yours or your eye doctor's. Of course, your doctor will help you decide whether or not it's time for your child to begin wearing contact lenses.

Is Your Child Ready for Contact Lenses?

Your child's motivation is key to his success in wearing contact lenses. He must be patient enough to master the skills of applying and removing lenses and be willing to take meticulous care of them.

Perhaps your child doesn't need to wear his glasses full time. If he can see fairly well without glasses, he may have less incentive to build the discipline it takes to wear and care for contact lenses. But if your child has to wear glasses full time and reaches the stage where he feels miserable about the way he looks, wearing contact lenses can help to polish a tarnished self-image.

Advantages of Wearing Contact Lenses

The light, compact design of contact lenses gives them many advantages over glasses. A contact lens is a thin, small, curved plastic disk that fits on the cornea, the clear outer covering of the eye in front of the colored part of the eye (iris) and the pupil. Because they ride on a tear layer on the front of the eye, contact lenses give your child a more accurate view of the world with less peripheral distortion than glasses.

When your child works up a sweat or goes out into the cold, his contact lenses won't fog up the way glasses do. Glasses for farsighted children tend to magnify objects, while glasses for nearsighted children make objects look smaller. Viewed through contact lenses, the world is normal size.

Children who wear glasses with a stronger prescription for one eye may have somewhat lopsided vision. Contacts will provide more balance in image size as well as improved depth perception and better ability to use both eyes together.

Because contact lenses provide better peripheral vision than glasses, they allow your child more freedom of movement. For young athletes, gymnasts, and dancers, wearing glasses might interfere with their performance. With contact lenses your child won't have to worry about glasses falling off in the heat of play or during a dramatic moment onstage. And thanks to the natural protection provided by the eyeball socket, contact lenses usually stay put.

Choosing the Best Contacts for Your Child

When contact lenses were first introduced over fifty years ago, only hard lenses made of a rigid, durable plastic were available. Today there are more comfortable options. Herewith, a roundup of contact lens options to consider.

Soft Contact Lenses

These tiny disks of water-loving plastic are often an excellent choice for youngsters. Made of a flexible material that absorbs water, soft contacts fit comfortably on the eye. This also makes it difficult for dirt and debris to get under the lens.

Another plus: soft contact lenses stay in place so that there's less chance of your child's losing them. And should your child accidentally dislodge the lens or rub it out of place, it won't harm his eye. Soft contact lenses allow oxygen to reach the cornea, which is important for eye comfort. Adjustment time: about two weeks.

Daily wear soft lenses require the most care of all soft lenses. Because they need to be removed every day for a thorough cleaning and disinfecting routine, daily wear soft lenses pose less threat of infection.

Daily wear soft lenses also need a weekly enzyme treatment. This solution removes the stubborn protein deposits that build up on lenses and which can cloud vision. (The natural protein found in tears bonds with contact lens material.) In some cases, this protein can harbor bacteria and irritate the eyes.

Extended wear soft lenses, meant to be left in the eyes overnight, are designed to be worn up to one week as prescribed by the doctor. They should be cleaned and disinfected when removed and given an enzyme treatment once a week.

Extended wear soft lenses allow the eyes to receive more oxygen than daily wear soft lenses. However, the odds of getting a corneal infection are greater for any individual who wears extended wear soft lenses. This is often the result of haphazard handling or improper cleaning and disinfecting. Many eye doctors recommend that extended wear lenses never be worn overnight.

Disposable soft lenses are also worn up to seven days, as prescribed by your doctor, then tossed out and replaced with a fresh pair. This regimen provides less chance of protein buildup and no hassle of weekly enzyme treatments. If your child loses one contact lens, you always have a new lens ready.

However, many doctors discourage the idea of prescribing disposable lenses for children if they are left in the eyes overnight. "Keep in mind that *any* contact lens is a foreign body in the eye," says pediatric ophthalmologist John Flynn, M.D. "If the lens is left in the eye improperly or the surface of the eye doesn't get enough oxygen, it can lead to an infection, scarring, or an ulcer."

And according to optometrist Julie Ryan, O.D., associate professor at Southern California College of Optometry, disposable contact lenses are often not an appropriate fit for young children under the age of six or seven.

If the convenience of disposable lenses appeals to you and your doctor approves them, the lenses *can* be removed at night, rubbed with a multipurpose cleansing and disinfecting solution, and kept in their storage case overnight.

Toric soft lenses, especially designed for people with astigmatism, can be worn by some children. Until they were developed, the irregular shape of the cornea of the astigmatic eye made it difficult for anyone with astigmatism to wear soft contacts, which move and turn on the eye because of the misshapen cornea. Toric lenses are designed to stay in place without moving or rotating on the eye and can also correct nearsightedness and farsightedness that may occur in combination with astigmatism.

In optometrist Julie Ryan's opinion, many children are not ready for toric soft lenses until the age of nine or ten or older. To make sure the lens won't rotate on the eye, the child has to sit through a long fitting session as different lenses are tried on and tested for accuracy. Unless your child is highly motivated, this process may be too tedious.

Which soft lens is best for *your* child? Your eye doctor knows best and will guide your choice. However, it may interest you to know that according to the Bausch & Lomb InVision Institute, 65 percent of all soft contact lens users (including young people under eighteen years of age) opt for daily wear lenses, and 15 percent choose extended wear lenses. Fewer than 5 percent of all contact lens users wear disposables.

Rigid "Hard" Contact Lenses

Although they are rarely prescribed today, even for adults, much less for children, these may be prescribed for your child if sharp, clear vision cannot be achieved with soft lenses.

Why are hard contact lenses initially less comfortable than soft lenses? They are made of a durable plastic material that keeps the cornea of the eye from getting a direct supply of oxygen. Instead, the eye receives oxygen indirectly; each time the eye blinks, the lens moves and the oxygen dissolved in the tears reaches the cornea. It takes about four to six weeks to build up tolerance and to adjust to a reduced supply of oxygen and reduced sensitivity of the cornea.

As for care, hard lenses need daily cleaning and disinfecting.

Rigid Gas-permeable Contact Lenses

These semihard lenses offer the optical clarity of hard lenses with less discomfort. Made of plastics combined with other materials such as silicone, gas-permeable lenses are almost as sturdy as hard contacts, but they are healthier for the eye.

Gas-permeable lenses "breathe" better than hard contacts, allowing the eye to get a direct supply of oxygen. (When eyes are deprived of oxygen they can swell, redden, and become sensitive to light.) It also takes less time (two to four weeks) to build up tolerance to gas-permeable lenses than hard contact lenses.

Children as young as three to four years of age may be good candidates for gas-permeable lenses, particularly if they show progressive nearsightedness. Gas-permeable lenses help slow the progression of myopia.

A daily cleaning and disinfecting routine plus a weekly enzyme cleaning is also a must for gas-permeable lenses. They are available as daily wear and as extended wear lenses.

Replacing Contact Lenses

Just as you toss out your child's toothbrush every three months to keep his teeth and gums healthy, you also need to have your child's contact lenses replaced on a regular basis. Even routine cleaning cannot completely remove the buildup of natural tear protein that accumulates on lenses.

While your child may not be able to see the film of protein on his lenses, he will be able to feel it. His eyes may feel red, itchy, or irritated, or his lenses may begin to feel uncomfortable. He may blink more frequently, have mucous on the eye, or complain of not being able to see as well.

Depending on changes in your child's vision, rigid contact lenses are replaced every one to three years. Disposable soft lenses are replaced with fresh lenses every week. And it is now recommended that daily wear and extended wear soft lenses be replaced at intervals of one month, three months, six months, or one year. The benefits of fresh lenses for your child: clear, sharp vision, more comfort, and healthy eyes.

TLC for Contact Lenses

Once your child is the proud owner of contact lenses, it is critical that he learn how to take meticulous care of them. While your doctor will provide your child with the proper guidelines, you can be his coach in making sure that he doesn't break training! The following tips will help.

- Make sure that your child keeps up with his daily and weekly cleansing routines. Dirty lenses can lead to infections and cause serious damage. Don't use tap water to clean contact lenses.
- Do remind your child to wash his hands with a mild nonperfumed soap before handling his contact lenses. Special optical soap is available.

- Be certain that your child reads package instructions and understands them before using contact lens products. Checking expiration dates is a must!
- Tell your child that if he loses one lens he should not throw away the other. It is less expensive to replace one lens than a pair!
- Advise your child to keep his nails short and filed smoothly. Long nails or nails with rough edges can easily scratch or tear lenses during removal and insertion.
- If your child likes to spritz on aerosol hair spray, deodorant, or cologne, remind her to do so *before* inserting lenses. (Opting for nonaerosol pump dispensers is a safer choice.)

SIGHT SAVERS: TIPS ON PREVENTING EYESTRAIN

Doing homework in dim light, playing video games or working on the computer for hours, sitting too close to the TV—all can put stress on your child's vision. Making the eyes work harder than they need to may cause eyestrain, headaches, tearing, or blurry vision. Your child may also complain that his eyes burn. To help your child learn how to be good to his eyes, try these tips from the American Optometric Association.

- To prevent eyestrain while your child is reading or doing homework, provide good overall room lighting as well as desk lighting. Fit the desk lamp with a shaded 100-watt bulb. Rule of thumb: desk lighting should be no more than three times brighter than overall room lighting. Make sure the desk lamp does not cast shadows on books or writing pages.
- Drapes, shades, or outside awnings help to soften glare from sunlight. Painting walls and (if practical) furnishings in soft, light colors with dull finishes to minimize reflected glare is also easy on your child's eyes.
- Show your child how to hold his book 12 to 16 inches away from his face. Both left and right pages should be kept at an

equal distance from your child's eyes, and the book should be tilted up to make it almost parallel to your child's face.
- Have your preschooler take a break from looking at picture books or watching television now and then. To help her shift her focus, have her walk into another room or gaze out the window.
- School-age children should give their eyes a rest from close-up work and TV viewing every hour. Focusing on distant objects for a few seconds helps.
- Encourage your child to sit up straight while reading, sitting at the computer, or watching TV. Focusing on objects at eye level helps to prevent fatigue.
- Discourage your child from reading or doing other close work in the car or other moving vehicle. If this is too difficult to enforce, make sure your child takes frequent breaks to look out the window.
- Teach your young computer whiz to tear herself away from the screen for a five-minute break every half hour. Adjust the screen brightness to three or four times the brightness of overall room lighting. And make sure there is no glare from windows or light reflection from lamps on the computer screen.
- Don't let your child watch TV in the dark. Each time your child looks away from the screen the pupils of his eyes dilate. Once he focuses on the TV screen again, the pupils constrict. This constant adapting is hard on the eyes. Instead, use soft overall lighting.
- Indirect or diffused lighting will prevent seeing the reflection of lamps on the screen. Make sure that you also adjust the screen's brightness and contrast controls for maximum eye comfort.
- The best viewing distance is at least five times the width of the television screen or at least six feet away from the set. (Sitting too close may strain the focusing muscles of the eyes.) And from this distance the image on the screen will appear sharper and clearer.

SAFETY ALERT: PREVENTING EYE INJURIES

Accidents can happen anywhere—at home, in school, on the playing field, or in your own backyard. To safeguard your child's eyes, you need to be on the alert for potential hazards. The following dos and don'ts from the American Academy of Ophthalmology will help keep your child's eyes safe.

> **Do** choose child-safe toys and games that are appropriate for your youngster's age. Be certain your child can handle his playthings with ease and confidence.
>
> **Don't** allow your child to play with projectile toys such as darts or bows and arrows.
>
> **Do** supervise your child when she handles sharp or pointy items such as pencils, scissors, and pen knives. Show her the safe way to use them.
>
> **Don't** permit your child to play with BB guns, air-powered rifles, and pellet guns. These are not toys but dangerous weapons. In fact, they are classified as firearms and can no longer be found in toy departments.
>
> **Do** keep all chemicals and sprays (including hair spray, room freshener, household cleaners, and fragrances) well out of reach of small children.
>
> **Don't** let your child play with paper clips, rubber bands, wire coat hangers, elastic cords, and fishing hooks. One false move could do serious harm to your child's eyes.
>
> **Don't** allow your child to play with fireworks—not even sparklers or small firecrackers—or to be anywhere in the vicinity of others who are setting them off. All fireworks are potentially dangerous.
>
> **Don't** let your child play in the yard while you're mowing the lawn. The moving blades can throw stones into the air, causing serious harm.
>
> **Do** insist that your child wear protective eyewear when playing

in dangerous sports such as racquetball, hockey, or baseball or when participating in workshops or chemistry lab.

Do be a good example. Wear protective eyewear whenever you use power tools, operate a rotary mower or line lawn trimmer, or hammer on metal.

FIRST AID FOR EYE INJURIES

If your child does suffer an eye injury, it is important that you get medical help right away. Even if the damage seems minor, you need to take your child to the eye doctor or your family physician immediately. (It's not always easy to tell at a glance the extent of the injury.) If your doctor is not available, bring your child to the nearest hospital emergency room. Prompt action can help to save your child's sight.

Until your child can get medical attention, it pays to know how to treat eye injuries with proper first aid care. Do remember that first aid is not a cure, but the first step in treating your child's injury and keeping it from getting worse. It does not take the place of medical treatment. The following guidelines will help you cope.

Removing Specks in the Eye

We all know that a tiny speck in the eye can feel like a boulder. This can be especially distressful for a small child. To prevent any speck or particles of dirt or sand from scratching the cornea, do not rub the eye. Instead, gently pull the upper lid over the lower lid. This will cause extra tearing to occur. Tell your child to blink a few times. This should dislodge the speck. If it doesn't, you might try rinsing the eye with tap water. Or squeeze a thin stream of a nonstinging balanced salt solution (available in pharmacies) into the corners of your child's eye. (Similar in composition to natural tears, the solution is more soothing than tap water.) After rinsing your child's eyes, have her blink a few more times.

If these strategies don't work or you're having a tough time getting a distressed child to sit still while you attempt to remove the speck, get medical help. Your doctor will use special anesthetic drops to numb the outside of the eye before removing the speck or particle.

Also, once the speck is out, you want to make sure your child doesn't have a scratched cornea, which can be quite painful. Have your child's eye checked by the doctor if she seems irritable, rubs her eyes, or shuns bright light.

Treating Chemical Burns

If a hazardous spray or chemical substance gets into your child's eyes, rinse them immediately with cool water. (If your child wears contact lenses, flush the eye first, then remove lenses.) Flood your child's eyes with water for at least fifteen minutes. Using your fingers to keep your child's eyes open as wide as possible, use a clean container to pour water into his eyes. (Do not use an eye cup.) Or hold his head under the faucet. Tell your child to roll his eyes as much as possible to help rinse out the chemicals. Once you've finished rinsing, do not bandage the eye. Take your child to your doctor or emergency room immediately.

Soothing a Blow to the Eye

If your child suffers a blow to the eye, apply first aid and then get to the eye doctor immediately. (Blurry vision or a black eye are signs that your child may have internal eye damage.) To reduce pain and swelling, apply an ice pack for about fifteen minutes. (A plastic bag filled with crushed ice will do.) Cold will also constrict the blood vessels, which helps to minimize any internal bleeding.

Treating Cuts of the Eye and Lid

Any cut of the eye or lid needs immediate medical care. To protect the injured eye, gently bandage it with a sterile pad and rolled gauze; lightly tape it into place. Do not rub the eye or apply pressure to the injured area, which can aggravate the injury. And do not rinse out your child's eye or try to remove any object lodged in the eye or lid. There's always the chance that your well-intentioned attempts can make the cut worse. Cuts can cause serious damage—any treatment must be left to medical specialists.

If there is a puncture wound to the eye, place a clean Dixie cup over the eye, tape it in place, and get to the emergency room. Once your child is old enough to follow instructions, teach him the above first-aid steps in case of emergency. He should also know to inform you immediately of his injury. If the accident happens away from home, instruct your child to promptly inform another adult such as a teacher or coach.

After your child's eye injury has healed, play it safe and have your child's eyes checked by a doctor. The injury may have caused a change in your child's vision. Proper testing will let you know whether your child needs additional treatment or corrective glasses or contact lenses.

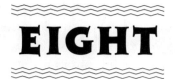

EIGHT

Clothes-Smart: Year-Round Guide to No-Fuss Dressing

A FEW YEARS AGO I produced a beauty story for *Parents* magazine that featured a young mother of six children, ages four to eleven. When our photography crew arrived at her home we found that Mom had her two sons and four daughters all decked out in matching crisp denim overalls and sunny yellow sweatshirts. They looked adorable!

But before the first photo was snapped, the photographer had another idea. "Hey, kids," he yelled. "Why don't you go back in the house and put on your favorite clothes. Wear whatever you want!"

The children were ecstatic. Inwardly I groaned. I thought my picture-perfect photo opportunity had been blown. A few minutes later the children tumbled down the stairs in a motley array of mismatched gear, including a faded red football jersey, a crumpled hot pink felt cap, purple nylon sweats with sports logos topped with a dressy blouse and golden locket, and an assortment of lived-in, grass-stained T-shirts. The color-coordinated, neat-as-a-pin perfection of the overalls and sweatshirts was gone. But the children beamed, and the group photo of this happy family remains one of my all-time favorites.

The lesson: children have powerful feelings about what they wear that may have nothing to do with an adult sense of style and taste. Choosing their own clothes is one way children learn to express personal style and to exercise some control in their well-ordered lives. It also teaches self-reliance.

This chapter is not about how to turn your child into a junior fashion victim. However, it can help you to make sure that the clothes in your child's closet are tops in comfort and quality. There are basics for building your child's wardrobe, choosing flattering clothes in all sizes and styles, tips on dressing for the weather, and a guide to stress-free shopping. On these pages you will also find ways to help your child master the skills of dressing himself as well as a game plan for ending early-morning dawdling and last-minute hunts for missing shoes.

If you take a relaxed approach to clothing and keep your child's comfort zone in mind, you can't go wrong. Now, that's being clothes-smart!

BABY'S FIRST WARDROBE

With the birth of your first child you sail into the unknown waters of buying children's clothing. Words such as "onesie," "stretchie," and "receiving blanket" will creep into your vocabulary as you learn the lingo of the layette.

When putting together baby's first wardrobe you want the fabrics that touch your baby's delicate skin to be soft. You want apparel designed to make diaper changing go quickly and smoothly. And from a fashion point of view, you may want bold colors and bright prints along with the traditional sweet pastel shades of yellow, pink, blue, and mint green. The following is a collection of what the well-dressed newborn should have at hand.

- 3 side-snap undershirts, 100 percent cotton, size three months
- 4–8 side-snap undershirts, 100 percent cotton, sizes six and twelve months
- 3–6 drawstring gowns (one size fits all, up to size nine months)
- 4–6 short- or long-sleeved bodysuits (a one-piece undershirt with a snap crotch; also called a "onesie"), sizes up to twenty-four months

- 4–6 creepers (a one-piece crotch-snap garment with buttons or snaps and no legs; to be worn as playwear in spring or summer) in 100 percent cotton or cotton blends. Or coveralls (a one-piece long-sleeved footless garment with legs; to be worn as playwear in fall or winter) in 100 percent cotton. Available with zippers, buttons, or snaps.
- 4–6 stretchies (a one-piece long-sleeved garment with legs and feet for round-the-clock wear) made of flame-retardant materials that meet the U.S. Consumer Product Safety Commission (CPSC) regulations for sleepwear. Available with zippers or snaps.
- 2–4 underwear sets (shirts with pants or bloomers)
- 1–2 cotton or acrylic cardigan sweaters
- 2–4 pairs of booties or socks
- 2–4 drooler bibs
- 1–2 cotton knit caps
- 4–6 receiving blankets in cotton, flannel, or cotton blend for swaddling the newborn
- 3–4 hooded terry cloth bath towels
- 3–4 baby washcloths
- 1–2 blanket sleepers (a one-piece long-sleeved zippered garment with legs and feet) for cold weather sleepwear
- 1 flame-resistant blanket

Buying Basics

When choosing among items with snaps, buttons, or zippers, consider this: Snaps and buttons may be more work. However, although zippers do get baby in and out of the garment quickly, they may catch on baby's skin. If you opt for zippers, easy does it!

To accommodate baby's diaper, one-piece items with legs, such as stretchies, need to be roomy from crotch to neck. Make sure the length is longer than the body. Drop shoulders and raglan sleeves allow little arms more freedom of movement.

Coveralls also come in footed styles for cozy winter wear. Those made of warm fabric such as fleece are sometimes called rompers or jumpsuits.

When putting together baby's layette, include items that are one or two sizes larger than baby's current weight. This allows room for growth. Because newborns grow so quickly, they'll speed through the three-months sizes in no time. Buy fewer things in this size and more of the six-months sizes.

The best bibs for newborns are made of soft terry cloth and are secured with snaps, ties, or Velcro. You can also find ribbed bibs that slip over baby's head. When baby is ready for solid foods, switch to a colorful plastic bib. Great for catching spills, it also washes clean quickly.

Pass up booties with attached decorations for plainer styles. Any item that baby can pull off and put in her mouth is a choking hazard.

Sleepwear Safety Tip

Parents who've discovered the comforts of cotton for themselves want to have clothing in this skin-soothing natural fiber for their babies. However, cotton is not a safe choice for sleepwear because it ignites easily. According to the CPSC, most fire tragedies that involve children occur when they are in their pajamas.

While it is more likely that a toddler helping Mom or Dad fix breakfast at the stove is at greater risk than an infant asleep in her crib, the CPSC regulations require that manufacturers make clothing sold as sleepwear with flame-retardant fabrics. For this reason, stretchies come in flame-retardant polyester knit or cotton/synthetic terry cloth.

As protective and durable as these fabrics are, they do pill and stain easily. If you prefer all-cotton sleepwear, you can now get 100 percent cotton items that have been treated with flame-retardant chemicals. However, they're not always easy to find. And there's this question: why put a natural fiber next to baby's skin if it's treated with chemicals?

To date, the CPSC is considering revising its sleepwear regulations as it pertains to close-to-the-body cotton sleepwear. They pose less of a safety hazard than flowing, loose-fitting cotton sleepwear, which ignites more easily.

CLOTHES YOU CAN COUNT ON

From the time they're toddlers right through the preteen years, children can get a lot of mileage from a collection of basics such as jeans,

T-shirts, and sweats. Basics can be dressed up or down, mixed and matched, or worn in layers for cozy comfort.

What else makes a piece of clothing a basic? Your child can slip into and out of it with ease (no tugging, or fumbling with fancy closures). The fabric is durable, can take the abuse of rough-and-tumble play, and comes clean in your washing machine. Thanks to the simple cut of most basics, they're unisex. This can certainly help to stretch a brother and sister's wardrobe—my brother Bob and I wore each other's sunsuits when we were toddlers—at least until they become more possessive about clothes.

Since the construction and fabric hold up so well, your child will probably outgrow a basic before he outwears it. And because a basic has more to do with function than fashion, it will never go out of style. The result: basics make great hand-me-downs. With a wardrobe built around basics, you don't have to shop so much as restock. Basics are also easy to put together, which helps your child to master the task of dressing himself. Herewith, a list of basics your child can grow on.

T-shirts

T-shirts are part of every child's basic uniform. Cotton tees are the most comfortable because they "breathe" and feel soft against tender skin. Cotton/poly blends are more durable, less prone to wrinkle, won't shrink in the dryer, and tend to cost less.

For newborns (sizes 0–3 months and 6–9 months) and infants (size 12 months), OshKosh B'Gosh makes T-shirts with snaps at the shoulder to make dressing a breeze. Tugging a T-shirt over the head can be frustrating for a toddler or for a preschooler who is learning to dress himself. Stretchy necklines solve the problem.

T-shirts also lend themselves to endless possibilities for expressing personal style and artistic whim. You can dye them, or paint your own designs with nontoxic fabric paints.

Jeans

For rough-and-tumble wear, nothing beats a pair of denim blue jeans, and the softer and more faded, the better. Jeans are hits not only with school-age children but with toddlers as well. You can even buy infant-size denims!

To speed up diaper changing, there are snap-crotch jeans for sizes up to 24 months by OshKosh B'Gosh. Their classic overall is also available with a snap crotch in sizes up to 4–T.

Jeans are versatile. You can get jeans with pockets lined in neon fabric, splashy paisley prints, slim-fit or baggy cuts, stonewashed, or studded with rhinestones. But not all jeans are created equal. Here's how to spot a quality pair of jeans.

- All-cotton denim is cooler to wear in hot, humid weather because it "breathes," allowing air and moisture to escape. Durable cotton/polyester blends are better for cooler weather.
- Look for straight seams. Twisted seams can feel uncomfortable. Make sure the stitching doesn't deviate from the seam line, which can weaken the seam.
- Elastic-waisted jeans are the most comfortable for infants and toddlers. Preschoolers will feel great in jeans designed with elastic at the back of the waist—they have the authentic look of grown-up jeans in front but are less confining.
- Velcro closures may be easier to manage than snaps or button fronts for children under five. Velcro can attach itself to other items of clothing in the wash, so be sure to secure closures before laundering.
- Check the fit. There should be ample room in the seat and legs. Make sure that the "rise," the distance between the crotch and waistline, is long enough.

Sweats

Sweatshirts and sweatpants are another big favorite with kids. Sweats in acrylic and polyester fabrics are great buys, but they also pill and stain easily. And as your child grows, you may need to replace them more often. (Bargain sweats have elastic cuffs that can't be rolled up.)

However, because they're lighter than the pricey high-quality sweats, they're perfect for warm weather.

Sweats made of 100 percent cotton and cotton/polyester blends are about double the price of bargain sweats, but you do get extra wear and high quality. As a rule, more expensive sweats are cut more generously. The fabric won't pill or lose its softness with wear and washing. Many are available with rib-knit cuffs. This allows you to start out with sweats that are one size too big and then roll up the sleeves and legs until your child grows into the size. And that means more wear for your money!

Leggings

Kids live in leggings. Because they hug the body, leggings are designed for action. And there are no snaps, zippers, or buttons for little fingers to wrestle with. The best are made of cotton with a touch of stretchy Lycra for extra give.

You can put leggings under a child's snowsuit or sweats for extra warmth. Boys and girls alike can wear leggings as lightweight alternatives to sweatpants. And girls can wear leggings under dresses or skirts for a trendy—and toasty—layered look, or under roomy oversize T-shirts.

IF YOUR CHILD TAKES A LARGE SIZE

Overweight youngsters have special needs. For instance, pants that are big enough to fit the waist may be too long. This means more work for you, as the legs need to be shortened. But in many cases the rise (the distance between the crotch and waist) is too long, and hemming won't fix that problem. Sleeves need to be amply cut but shoulders shouldn't droop. And waistbands should be comfortable but secure.

Fortunately, today you *can* find clothing especially designed for youngsters who take large sizes. One excellent resource is Kids at Large, a catalog that specializes in playwear and school clothes for boys and girls from 55 pounds to 285 pounds. (Large-size kids are at least 20 percent over their ideal weight.) To order a catalog, call 1-617-769-8575.

A look at the latest large-size clothes will show you that kids today don't have to give up fashion for fit. The current crop come in hot neon colors as well as splashy prints and spiffy skateboard patterns. For flattering clothes that fit, check for the following details.

- Shop for pants and shorts with all-elastic multineedled waistbands for extra give. While large-size jeans often have elastic waistbands in back, all-elastic-waist jeans are now available.
- Dress pants and casual pants cut wide and full in the seat and thigh with a gently tapered leg are a good choice. This cut allows for roomy fit where needed and creates a slimming silhouette.
- Turtlenecks should have a relaxed fit and extra length—no tight squeezes at the neck! Tops with dropped shoulders and extra room under the arm allow arms more freedom of movement.
- Dresses with dropped waists are comfortable, delightfully feminine, and flatter the hip area. Gentle V-necks or softly scooped necklines create the illusion of a longer, leaner line.
- For girls, a one-piece swimsuit in a jazzy tropical color with a contrasting diagonal insert in black seems to make the tummy disappear. Flirty ruffles are also pretty camouflage.
- Baggy boxer-style trunks with a drawstring waist in neon-bright surfer colors put boys in the swim in style.
- If your youngster wants to show his stripes, opt for vertical rather than horizontal stripes. They draw the eye down to make him look leaner. Small prints such as dots and confetti patterns help to minimize a middle.

STRESSLESS DRESSING

Does this sound familiar? It's seven A.M. and the morning rush clock is ticking. You want your daughter to wear the sweater Grandma knitted for her last birthday to a family gathering, but she's stubbornly holding out for the same sweatshirt she's been wearing for the last five days. Your son can't find his sneakers, and his socks are mismatched.

No parent wants to begin the day arguing with a child over what to wear. But there is a better way to get your child ready for the day that is easier on both you and your child. The following game plan will help.

Get Organized!

To put an end to hectic mornings, lay out clothing the night before. Come up with two choices of outfits and let your child take his pick. This will allow your child to exercise some decision-making power, which is half the battle in getting young children dressed.

Be Ready for the Weather

Searching for umbrellas or mittens when you're in an early morning fog is not the best way to start your day. Listen to the weather report at night, and locate any special outerwear your child may need for the morning.

Pin mittens or gloves to coat sleeves, zip in the lining of a raincoat, attach the detachable hood to a winter jacket, ferret out rain boots or snow boots, slip a scarf in the sleeve of a coat. Being a step ahead of foul weather can put a little sunshine in your day!

Cure for the Wigglies

It's tough to dress a toddler or preschooler who fusses and fidgets. My own mom's remedy for this is to create distractions. Using your imagination, she says, is easier than trying to convince a child to sit still. Sing a nonsense rhyme or a favorite song. Talk about the fun you're going to have that day. Make funny faces. Once you're the center of your child's attention, you can zip through the steps of dressing him without a hitch. If you can't pin down your toddler to put on his shoes and socks, leave them off until he's in his high chair for breakfast. While he eats you can quickly slip them on.

Bringing a Dawdler up to Speed

If your child is old enough to dress herself but seems to move in slow motion or fits and starts, she may be trying to tell you something. Perhaps all the rushing around in your house makes her feel anxious, and she copes by daydreaming or dressing at her own comfortable pace. Or perhaps your child knows that once she's dressed, you'll soon be off and running to work.

One way to take the pressure off is to set your alarm clock a little earlier—not so easy if you're not a morning person, but early rising may be worth the effort. It will help to give you extra quality time to spend with your child, which can be very reassuring to him or her.

Is your child's clothing designed to make dressing go quickly? Overalls with two-button straps are easier to handle than hook-and-slide adjustable straps. Pullover tops take less time to put on than those with buttons and snaps. Elasticized waists make pants, shorts, and skirts easy to pull on and off. (My four-year-old nephew, Matthew, loves his sneakers with Velcro closures because he doesn't have to wait for Mom to tie his shoelaces.) When your child can put himself together without struggling with complicated fastenings, it will give him a wonderful sense of achievement and independence.

Have a contest: "Can you put on your shoes and socks by the time I count to ten?" "Can you get dressed faster than Daddy?" Such strategies can motivate a child who can't resist a challenge. Making dressing a first step in a routine can also help a dawdler to get going. "As soon as you're dressed, we'll read a story." "If you're dressed in time for breakfast, we'll play your new music cassette."

More Help

Make sure that clothing is within easy reach. Stack clothes on bottom shelves, or keep them in bottom drawers. Covered wire closet cubes with child-height hanging racks are also handy. See-through plastic drawers for shoes and sweaters make these items easy to find—they store easily on closet shelves. And to keep your child's sock and underwear drawer from being a jumbled mess, you might want to invest in clear plastic sock boxes that fit inside a drawer.

Last, accept reality gracefully. Some days dressing will go smoothly and some days you'll lose it. But the more provoked you become, the more stressful dressing becomes. If a cranky toddler resists your best efforts, ask your partner for help. When your household is in an uproar, dress your child in a quiet room. And if an older child continually rejects your clothing choices, talk about it. You may be surprised at the cooperation a little open discussion can bring!

BUNDLE UP!
CHILL-CHASING CLOTHES FOR WINTER

'Tis the season for ice skating and sledding, making frosty snow angels, and warming up with steamy mugs of hot cocoa. With the first cold snap you start to pile on the winter clothes—sweaters, snowsuit, mittens, scarf, boots, hat, the works!

One hour later, your child is a zippered-up, well-wrapped bundle who can barely walk out the door to play. Or you may have an older child who insists he doesn't feel Jack Frost nipping at his nose and goes out into the cold sans hat and gloves. The trick to comfortable winter dressing is to put your child in clothes that hold in body heat without adding extra bulk—and without making him look silly!

Dressing your child in layers keeps her warm by trapping insulating air between the pieces of clothing. As the temperature drops, you can always add layers. Once your child is indoors or works up a sweat outdoors, you can easily peel off the layers as needed.

Making Baby Cozy

You want to take steps to protect your baby against exposure to cold and wind without overdressing her. Babies can easily become overheated—tender skin then breaks out in what is called midwinter prickly heat.

Most pediatricians advise that you dress your baby as warmly or lightly as you dress yourself. Keep in mind, though, that premature infants may need an extra layer or two. "Preemies" have less body fat than full-term babies to insulate body heat. And their ability to regulate body temperature isn't as efficient. Basic layers for babies include the following.

- A soft long-sleeved undershirt
- A pair of tights
- A shirt
- A light-to-medium-weight nonscratchy sweater
- Toddler-size thermal socks over cotton socks
- Mittens (the thermal socks can also double as mittens)
- A warm, snug-fitting hat that covers baby's ears but not her eyes. (Most body heat is lost through the head via the unprotected blood vessels in the scalp.) Try a funnel-shaped knitted pullover hood. It also keeps baby's neck warm and can't be tugged off by little fingers.
- A waterproof or water-repellent snowsuit. (Look for machine-washable snowsuits.)

A modern alternative to the traditional snowsuit is the Baby Bag®. This loose, footed garment is designed without sleeves, which speeds up dressing baby. You simply slip your little one into the Baby Bag®, zip it up, and pull the drawstring. Your bundle of joy is free to move her arms inside or outside the garment. Ideal for infants, the Baby Bag® is also available for older babies and toddlers up to two years. You can order it through mail order catalogs.

Layering for Toddlers and Up

For older children, the rules for layering are similar to those for babies. Keep in mind that a preschooler won't always tell you when he's too cold or overdressed and a school-age child can drive you up with the wall with her insistence that she wear light layers on a blustery day.

Some kids don't get as chilled as others; they can defy the North Wind in unzipped jackets and not catch cold. If you're concerned that your child doesn't dress warmly enough, discuss it with your pediatrician. In the meantime, follow these basic guidelines for coldproof layering.

Slip on a T-shirt or thermal underwear. You want a soft, absorbent fabric next to your child's skin. Consider cotton, polypropylene (an insulating synthetic), or silk (ski underwear often comes in body-warming silk). Add a turtleneck top, a flannel shirt, then a warm sweater. (Wool may be unbearably itchy for tender skin; opt for soft knits.) Top layers with a ski jacket or storm coat. (You can also layer a down vest underneath the jacket for extra warmth.)

Put tights plus thin cotton socks under thermal socks. Keep legs warm with sweatpants, cozy corduroy pants, or knitted leggings. (Blue jeans get stiff with the cold. Jeans also aren't warm enough for icy weather unless they're lined with flannel.) If your little girl opts for tights with her dress or skirt, add knitted leg warmers. Winterproof feet with sturdy, protective boots or shoes. Slip on snug-fitting gloves or glove liners under a roomier pair of mittens. Top off everything with a snuggly, nonscratchy scarf (make sure it's not too long) and a warm hat.

A Word about Winter Jackets

For keeping your child warm and comfortable, down-filled jackets have a lot going for them. The light weight of down feathers means less bulk to weigh upon your child. And down allows body moisture to evaporate, so that if your child works up a sweat he'll cool off quickly and won't feel damp and sticky. But keep in mind that down is expensive and is not easy-care. Yes, most down jackets today can be machine-washed. But you still need to lay them out flat to dry. Still, you may find down worth the price and extra care.

Although not as lightweight as down, polyester fiberfill does a good job of keeping kids warm. It also launders more easily and won't need reshaping to dry. Look for quilted linings that keep the polyfill from shifting. And make sure that the filling is not too flat.

When shopping for a winter jacket, look for a tag that indicates the garment is water-repellent. Many jackets today are treated with 3M Scotchguard, a rain and stain repellent. Multistitched elastic along the bottom helps to keep the wind out. So do knitted cuffs on sleeves.

Make sure drawstrings have preknotted nylon ends. This keeps the drawstring from unraveling and helps it to stay put. Opt for plastic zippers. (Metal zippers can catch on the skin and scratch or cut.) Look for wind flaps over the zipper. This feature helps to seal out icy gusts.

In Step with Winter Boots

Before your little one starts to walk she won't need a waterproof boot for snowy weather, but you still want to keep her feet warm. One option is a nonwalker baby boot such as Stride-Rite's "Spout." Made with a soft polyurethane upper, this boot has a cozy fleece lining to coldproof tiny toes. Velcro straps make the boots easy to put on and take off.

Once your child is romping through snowdrifts you'll want waterproof protection. (Waterproof materials keep water out. Water-resistant materials repel water, but if your child were to stand in a deep puddle, water could seep into the boot.) For sizes 1–4 and sizes 5–10 you can get a boot with a seamless foot made of waterproof PVC (polyvinyl chloride), a durable, flexible manmade material that won't stiffen up in the wet and cold. The foot of the boot is stitched with nylon to water-resistant uppers. A pile lining, which is smoother than fleece, warms up feet.

For children who take a size 9–4, Stride-Rite makes a waterproof boot called the Snow Bank. It has nylon cuffs and a drawstring to allow for a snug fit. The foam-filled brushed nylon inner sole is removable, so if it gets wet, you can slip it out to dry. And without the lining, the boot doubles as a rain boot. Whatever boot you buy for your child, make sure that the bottom of the outer sole has good traction to prevent spills on icy or slippery ground.

RAINY DAYS:
DRESS CODE FOR DOWNPOURS
AND DRIZZLES

Sloshing through puddles and twirling umbrellas are part of the unfettered joy of childhood. You want your child to have his rainy day fun, but you also want to keep him dry and comfortable. The following tips will help you to find protective rainwear that's sure to make a big splash with your kids.

Adult-size raincoats are often made of canvas and cotton, but this is not the fabric of choice for kids. The most widely used rainproof material is waterproof PVC vinyl. It comes in a shiny or matte finish. (Most kids, even up to sizes 7–14, love the shiny finish.) Other waterproof fabrics include Supplex nylon and Polyflex. All are flexible and won't stiffen up when the temperature drops. Water-resistant PVC vinyl is also available.

Linings create warmth and keep the material of the raincoat away from your child's skin. A thin cotton flannel lining turns a raincoat into a rain or shine coat for spring. A quilted flannel lining makes a raincoat warm enough to wear during the crisp days of fall. And a raincoat lined with polar fleece, a fuzzy, chill-chasing material, doubles as an all-weather winter coat, as long as temperatures aren't too cold. (Wippette Kids makes rainwear with a zip-out polar fleece lining.) With the change of seasons, zip-out linings have a way of disappearing. If you opt for rainwear with a removable lining, be sure to sew in your child's name tag. And put one in the raincoat, too!

Quality counts. Look for pockets that are stitched on rather than fused on. They should also be deep and roomy. Closures should be sturdy and secure. Snaps are a snap to do and undo. Zippers and buckles are also available. (Buckles are often more for show than function. Toddler-size coats come with snaps underneath the buckles.)

Corduroy collars keep the chill off your child's neck, and a hood protects the head. If the raincoat doesn't have a hood, invest in a wide-brimmed waterproof hat. Ties or a stretchy elastic band that fits under the chin will keep the hat in place even on a windy day.

The trendy anorak is now available as rainwear in water-repellent nylon. You can find them in sizes for children from three months up to twelve years of age. One excellent resource is the Hanna Andersson catalog. Call 1-800-222-0544.

Ponchos with hoods to slip over sweaters and jackets keep kids of all ages warm and dry in cool weather. They are also roomy enough to wear over a coat. For summer showers, you can pop on a poncho without a lining.

Your child will get more wear out of her raincoat if you buy one that's slightly larger than her size. To adjust the fit, roll up the sleeves. With the extra room you can layer tops and sweaters under the raincoat for extra warmth. Just make sure that the raincoat isn't so long that your child trips over it!

For puddle-proof rainboots, follow the guidelines for choosing snow boots (see page 184). However, unless the weather is cold, fleece lining will be too bulky. A light lining such as brushed nylon keeps feet warm as well as dry. Some rain boots, such as Stride-Rite's Two-Step cowboy boot for girls sizes 10–4, come with pull rings. These special rubber handles allow your child to pull on her boots by herself.

CHILL OUT! COOL SUMMER STYLE

It's summertime, the living is easy, and so is the approach to dressing. During my own childhood summers, my brothers and sisters and I lived in our bathing suits on the off-chance that we might be invited to swim in a neighbor's pool or persuade Dad to drive down to the Jersey shore. Besides, we loved the reckless freedom of running around wearing next to nothing.

Times haven't changed much, and kids will still take swimwear over more covered-up clothes any day. Luckily, you don't need much else to fill out your child's hot-weather wardrobe. A collection of T-shirts, shorts, bike pants, and (for girls) loose sundresses will see your child through the golden days of summer in style.

Clothes That Beat the Heat

Your child will feel cool and comfortable even on steamy, sultry days if you dress him in oversize, baggy clothes that allow air to circulate around his body. Loose-fitting shorts and unwaisted overalls held up by suspenders are two choices.

Choose lightweight fabrics that float away from the body. Good choices include gingham, seersucker, madras, calico, sheeting, lawn, and chambray. And when these fabrics are made with cotton, all the better.

Cotton is like air-conditioning for the body. Because it "breathes," it allows perspiration from the body to pass into the air. And as you wash and wear it, this natural fiber gets softer with time. More points for cotton: it doesn't build up a static charge, won't pill, and is hypoallergenic.

Clothes-Smart

All-cotton (100 percent) garments do shrink a bit after washing, but that doesn't necessarily mean that you have to buy clothing two or more sizes bigger. Ask the salesperson for the shrinkage rate of the garment.

Cotton/poly blends give you some of the comfort and breathability of cotton plus the durability of synthetic fiber. The higher the percentage of cotton in the garment (65 percent or more), the less it will pill in the wash. Whether you opt for all cotton or cotton blends, the following clothing choices will make summer dressing a breeze.

- Put your infant in a stretchy sleeveless or short-sleeve snap-crotch romper made of cotton jersey. Some come with covered elastic in the legs for a more comfortable fit. Also available in cotton blends.
- Cotton and cotton-blend pullover knit shorts with elasticized waistbands are great for toddlers and children sizes 4–7. Look for triple-stitched waistbands. Extra give means longer wear.
- Drop-waist sundresses in madras, gingham, and cotton sheeting keep little girls (sizes 4–6x) and big girls (sizes 7–14) looking and feeling fresh in a heat wave. Look for deep-cut necklines and armholes to allow for "air-conditioning."
- Breezy pullover trapeze tops and flyaway sleeveless tops in cotton knit, also for big girls and little girls, swing away from the body for light and airy comfort.
- Cotton denim bib overalls in colorful stripes are the perfect summer uniform for kids. You can put your child in this indestructible easy-care basic starting with infant sizes up to little boy sizes 4–7.
- For toddler boys up through preteens, the baggy "hang-ten" surfer look is in! One must-have: pull-on cotton surfer pants with side pockets, in wild prints.

Make Waves!
Swimwear That's Fun to Wear

For your daughter you want a swimsuit that won't stretch out after a few wears and that stays up whether she's building sand castles or competing in her first swim meet. Antron/Lycra, cotton/Lycra, nylon/Lycra, and polyester/Lycra have two-way stretch. That is, they stretch both vertically and horizontally.

The Lands' End catalog offers swimsuits for girls with zigzag stitching at the armholes, neck, and leg openings that gives with every move your child makes. To order the catalog call 1-800-356-4444.

The cut of your daughter's suit should be generous enough to cover her bottom. To make sure the suit stays up, choose one with T-back straps cut around the shoulders. Other good choices are crisscrossed straps and adjustable straps.

Baby and toddler girls who are still in diapers can wear a bloomer-style suit. This is a tank-top style with bubble-shaped legs roomy enough to accommodate diapers.

For boys from toddlers through the preteen years who love the California surfer look, there are loose-fitting jams—baggy, above-the-knee-length shorts with wide legs and an adjustable drawstring waist. There are also knee-knocker surfer pants and mid-thigh-length drawstring trunks.

Because sitting in wet trunks feels "yucky," swimsuits made of quick-drying fabrics such as a cotton/polyester blend are a must. Trunks made of 100 percent Supplex nylon beat cotton/poly blends in drying time, yet breathe like cotton and feel just as light and comfortable against the skin.

Fun at Your Feet: Summer Shoes for Kids

When your child's not running barefoot she'll want to wear shoes that make her feel light on her feet. Canvas slip-on sneakers with rubber soles are a shoo-in for boys and girls of all ages. Styles are available in prewalker sizes 1–4 as well as sizes 5–10 and 11–3. One style to look for has a stretchy T-strap for slip-proof fit. These are a great alternative to plain slip-on sneakers for small children who may slip out of this style if the shoe gaps at the heel.

Sturdy sandals come in soft leathers and water-resistant synthetics such as PVC vinyl. (Manmade materials are easy to wipe clean.) Double straps allow for secure fit. For little feet (sizes 5–10) you can

Clothes-Smart

also find PVC vinyl sandals with Velcro closures. There are also sandals with snap closures.

Most kids I know love to kick up their heels in colorful plastic and vinyl jellies. (I'm sure the squishy feeling is part of the appeal.) Keep in mind that plastic and vinyl can't breathe to let heat escape. There's also no absorbent lining to soak up moisture as your child's feet perspire. If possible, try to convince your youngster to wear socks with her jellies to prevent blisters. Or reserve them for beach and pool wear only.

The bottom soles of all kids' summer shoes should be slip-proof. Soles made of PVC vinyl are very durable. And soles made of EVA (ethylene vinyl acetate, a light, flexible thermoplastic), blown rubber, or vulcanized rubber are lightweight as well as flexible. Pebbled or textured surfaces also have extra grip.

HOW-TOS FOR HASSLE-FREE SHOPPING

When it comes to buying your child's clothes, you don't want to shop till you drop. You want to get in and out of the store, pronto, with exactly what your child needs. You don't want to pay a fortune. To fine-tune your own shopping system, try these tips from the fashion editors of *Parents* magazine.

- Go through your child's closet and note what items are worn out or too small. Make a list of what your child needs. (To avoid impulse buys, stick to your list!)
- Check the prices for the items on your list with the same items sold at better retail stores. Compare them with the prices marked at your favorite bargain center. This will help you to recognize a good deal.
- You'll save 75 percent off retail if you shop at the end of the season. Fall and winter clothes are a steal in February; May is bargain month for spring items; and July is the best time for summer sales.
- Do you prefer to shop at the start of the season? Special holiday promotions help you to save big bucks. For example, you

can get great bargains on spring clothes around President's Day in mid-February.
- If your kids hate to shop, go alone. As long as you're shopping for basics in colors and styles you know your kids like (and in sizes that fit), they can try them on at home.
- If you have a picky dresser it may be easier to bring him along. But do go to the store ahead of time and scope out several outfits for him to try on when you return to shop.
- Before you plunk down your money, check the store's policy on returns. If it's a sale item you may not get a refund, or you may get a sales credit.

How to Spot Value

Quality counts. You don't want to spend your hard-earned money on children's clothing that falls apart after a few spins in the washing machine. What makes an item of clothing a great buy: good fabric such as soft cotton knits and acrylic blends, and durable denim, flannel, and corduroy; expert tailoring (well-sewn seams, roomy cuts, ample armholes to allow for layering); and attractive, well-made details such as secure buttons and snaps.

The following tips on construction details from Ernie Lippman, national product development manager of children's wear for Sears, will help you to zero in on good value.

- Examine buttons. Four-hole cross-stitched buttons are more tightly secured than straight-stitched buttons.
- No-rust, washable plastic zippers with a lock at the bottom or top won't catch or scratch like metal zippers. However, heavy fabrics such as denim jeans need metal zippers for hold. Plastic would be too lightweight.
- Pockets should be deep enough to stash a handful of your child's treasures. The top and bottom corners take the most stress and should be reinforced.
- Necklines should have a clean finish to prevent chafing. Cover-stitching or double-needling the neckline adds extra

strength. Tops such as T-shirts should be reinforced at the shoulder and neck.
- Multineedled waistbands snap back into shape with ease. Look for double-stitching on armholes and side seams. Opt for dresses and skirts with hems long enough to let out as your child grows.

FEET FIRST: TIPS ON SHOES

Parents have plenty of good questions about shopping for shoes: "Is leather always best? It's so expensive!" "What's the best time of day to shop for shoes?" "How can I make sure my child's shoes aren't too tight or too roomy?" "Athletic shoes are all the rage. But are they good for growing feet?"

To make sure the shoe fits and has your child stepping out in comfort, follow the upcoming guidelines.

Baby Shoes

When your toddler begins to take her first wobbly steps you become concerned with what kind of shoe she should wear. Actually, the more your child can go barefoot, the better.

Without the confinement of shoes, little toes can bend more easily. Your child's feet have more freedom of movement, which gives them a better chance to become strong and supple. Going shoeless also results in better balance, because bare feet can grip the floor more easily.

Of course, there are times when, for practical reasons, your baby will need shoes to protect her feet. The best shoes for baby are a step away from barefoot. For smart shoe shopping, follow these easy tips.

Make sure the shoe fits. Both of your child's feet should be measured by an experienced salesperson. If one foot is larger than the other, choose the fit for the larger foot. For the most accurate measurement, your child should be standing. Feet spread and elongate when bearing the full weight of your child. Feet need toe-wiggling room. Make sure that the shoes have about a thumb's width (¼ inch to ½ inch) from the end of the longest toe to the lip of the shoe. Check that the widest part of the shoe meets the ball of the foot (the widest part of the foot).

Have your child "road-test" his shoes in the store. His gait should be natural, close to that of his walk when he's barefoot. If not, the shoes may be too stiff. Next, take off your child's shoes and socks and check for any red marks or other signs of soreness, such as rubbed-off skin. If it looks as if the shoes are putting too much pressure on the feet, try another size or style.

Opt for lightweight, flexible materials. Good choices are canvas, suede, and leather. Check the soles of the shoe. The surface should be flexible. If soles are too hard, the shoes will cramp your toddler's gait. The sole should also grip the ground when your child walks. To make sure the sole neither slips nor catches, slide it along a smooth surface.

TIPS ON STYLE AND CONSTRUCTION FOR BABY SHOES

- High-tops help to keep baby's shoes on his feet. They also keep ankles warm. Because babies have such round, chunky feet, the contours of the heel haven't developed enough to hold low-cut shoes in place.
- Lace-up shoes are also more secure on baby's feet than slip-ons or shoes with buckles.
- Shoes with squared-off toes conform to the natural contours of baby's foot.
- Uppers should be stitched to the sole, not glued. This allows the shoe to move with the foot with more ease.
- A split-sole design keeps the front of the sole from sticking and allows the heel to grip the ground. This promotes a smoother heel-and-toe motion with every step.
- A molded toe prevents tumbles and tripping. (A protruding lip can catch on objects in your baby's path.) The material of the lining should be soft.

Note: If it's important for you to have a shoe endorsed by foot care experts, look for the American Podiatric Medical Association's

(APMA) Seal of Acceptance. This indicates that the shoes have met the APMA's current medical standards for quality and fit.

For Toddlers and Up: When Your Child Needs New Shoes

Keep in mind that as your child grows up, the same rules for checking fit for baby's shoes apply to older children as well. Before you know it, shoes that were a perfect fit for your child will become too small. (Fact: a child's shoe size can change thirty-four times before the age of ten!) Since children's feet grow at different rates (sometimes in spurts, sometimes more slowly), you need to do a routine check every few weeks.

You will also discover that your child may develop definite likes and dislikes concerning her footwear. My eleven-year-old niece, Anna, likes to show off her "pretty shoes" whenever possible, while her pals wear scruffy sneakers to school. Although you may have to compromise on matters of style and taste, you still want to make sure that your child wears quality shoes. The following tips will help.

Shop where the premium is put on service, not style. The salesperson should know how to measure your child's foot and test the shoe for proper fit. A salesperson should never try to push any shoe because "all the kids are wearing them."

While you want to give your child some opportunity to exercise her right to choose, don't give her full rein. She may zero in on shoes that don't fit properly. Instead, find two pairs that are a perfect fit and allow her to choose between the two.

Go shoe shopping in the afternoon rather than the morning. By midday your child's feet can swell up to half a size, especially in warm, humid weather. Keep this in mind when shopping for patent leather and other materials that are not especially pliant.

Sneakers with Velcro closures are a great time-saver, but they're not always best for every foot. Children with slender or narrow heels may slide around inside the shoe. Your child may need the support of lace-up shoes.

Shoes that feel good in the store may not actually wear well once your child gives them the full treatment (running, jumping, sliding, hopping) at home. For the first week or so, do a routine check of your child's feet at the end of the day. Look for any red areas or sore spots. If you suspect that the shoes are too tight, take them back to the store.

Choosing a Child's Athletic Shoe

Sports stars have made athletic shoes glamorous and a hot ticket among the savvy school-age set. (My nephews, Christopher, thirteen, and Adam, eight, wear their high-tops as dress shoes!) Since your youngster will probably spend more time in athletic shoes than any other type of footwear, you want to make sure that he wears shoes that are well built and designed for comfort and proper support. For a step in the right direction, try these tips from The Athlete's Foot.

Ask your pediatrician what to look for in an athletic shoe for your child. If the shoe fits properly, it can help to promote proper bone and muscle development. If your child has a medical problem related to flat feet or high arches, you may need to consult a podiatrist.

Several features promote internal stability. A contoured midsole allows the foot to sit down in the shoe. Fiberboards in the rear foot of the shoe allow for stability. An absence of fiberboard in the forefront allows for flexibility. For external support, the heel counter at the back of the shoe should be firm. High-tops and three-quarter cuts give feet extra support.

Midsoles made of compression-molded EVA, or polyurethane, a flexible manmade material, provide good cushioning. Outsoles made of rubber or polyurethane can take a lot of wear and tear. Look for stitched reinforcement in the toe area that can stand up to toe dragging.

SPILLS AND STAINS:
REMOVAL TIPS FOR STICKY SITUATIONS

Making messes is part of being a child. And it always seems as if the ketchup is spilled or the chocolate is smeared whenever kids are wearing their best clothes. Not to worry. The following handy tips will make light work of cleaning up spills and removing common stains.

But first a few words of friendly advice: Attend to spots and stains as soon as you notice them. The longer they sit, the harder it is to get them out. You should always try to remove the stain before you launder the soiled piece of clothing—washing it first can "set" the stain in the fabric. Heat also sets stains, so no hot water, please. For the same reason, you should never iron over a stain or toss a stained garment in the clothes dryer. And if the clothing isn't washable or is labeled "Dry clean only," bring it to the dry cleaner as quickly as you can; be sure to point out where the stain is so that the garment can be pretreated. Now, to the rescue, operation stain removal.

Ballpoint pen ink. Spritz the spot with hair spray and blot it with a dry, clean cloth. Repeat until ink fades. Or sponge on rubbing alcohol before washing it.

Blood. Soak the garment in cold water immediately. If the stain won't budge, try an enzyme presoak. After soaking, wash as usual. Another trick: Apply meat tenderizer or cornstarch and enough cool water to make a paste. After fifteen to thirty minutes, sponge off with cool water.

Chewing gum. Place an ice cube over the gum to harden it. Next, scrape it off with the edge of a dull knife. Last, stroke on an enzyme stain remover stick such as Spray 'n Wash Stain Stick.

Chocolate. Remove excess with a spoon or spatula. Apply club soda to stain, then soak garment in warm water with an enzyme detergent. Launder as usual.

Citrus juice. Put garment in warm water with enzyme presoak. After thirty minutes, rinse well and launder.

Crayon stains. Place the garment between sheets of clean paper towel or pieces of brown paper bag. Press with a warm iron. Replace the paper towels or bag as it absorbs crayon.

Cream and milk. Stroke on a stain remover stick. Next, wash with laundry detergent in cool water.

Grape juice. Treat stain with stain remover stick. Allow it to set for twenty-four hours. Launder as usual.

Grass stains. Apply rubbing alcohol, blotting up any excess. Sponge stain with water, then sponge it with dishwashing detergent. Rinse stain and launder it. Use bleach if fabric is durable enough for bleaching.

Grease. Place the garment with the stain facedown on clean paper towels. Using a clean, white cloth and liquid detergent, go over the back of the garment. Launder as usual.

Lipstick. Holding paper towels over the spot, apply a dry-cleaning solvent such as Carbona Spot Remover and work on the back of the fabric. Once the stain fades, dampen it and rub a bar of soap over it. For stubborn stains, apply a few drops of ammonia mixed with liquid soap; rinse well.

Makeup. Shake on a little talcum powder to absorb the oils found in face makeup. Soak clothing in warm water with detergent. Launder as usual.

Nail polish. Blot excess polish with a dry, clean cloth. Turn garment inside out and treat stain with a nonoily nail polish remover. (Place dry cloth underneath the garment to blot excess remover.) Rinse well and launder as usual. *Note:* Do not use polish remover on acetate or triacetate. Instead, scrape polish off with a blunt knife.

Water-base fingerpaint. This works only if the paint is still wet. Sponge off the paint with cool water, being careful not to spread the stain any further. Rinse well and launder. If the paint has dried, you may be able to scrape it off with the edge of a blunt knife.

Bibliography

Bacon, Kenneth H. "Coalition Pushes for Plumbing Device to Help Prevent Accidental Scaldings." *Wall Street Journal*, May 11, 1990.
Briggs, Dorothy Corkville. *Your Child's Self-Esteem*. New York: Doubleday, 1975.
Chase, Deborah. *The Medically Based No-Nonsense Beauty Book*. New York: Alfred A. Knopf, 1974.
Consumer Reports. "Blue Jeans." *1992 Buying Guide*, December 1991.
Di Grappa, Carol. "Bundle Up!" *Parents*, February 1990.
———. "Rain Dance." *Parents*, April 1991.
———. "Great Buys." *Parents*, March 1992.
Finkelstein, Alix. "Bathing Your Baby." *Parents*, June 1990.
———, ed. "Warning: Talc Can Be Toxic." *Parents*, February 1992.
Fitzpatrick, Jean Grasso. "Dressing Kids Without Stress." *Parents*, November 1990.
Flusser, Marilise. *Party Shoes to School and Baseball Caps to Bed*. New York: Fireside, 1992.
Furgason, Maija K., ed. "Rx for Sand in the Eye." *Parents*, August 1991.
Gewirtzman, Garry B., M.D. *Smooth as a Baby's Bottom*. Hollywood, Fla.: Frederick Fell Publishers, 1988.
Hales, Dianne. "Sure Ways to Break Nervous Habits You Hate." *Self*, February 1988.
Haberman, Fredric, M.D., and Denise Fortino. *Your Skin*. New York: Berkley Publishing, 1987.

Bibliography

Israeloff, Roberta. "Hello, World!" *Parents*, November 1990.
Karlsrud, Katherine, M.D., and Dodi Schultz. "Overdoing by Overdressing." *Parents*, November 1990.
———. "Minor Bumps and Tumbles." *Parents*, August 1991.
———. "Keeping Your Baby Clean." *Parents*, February 1992.
Katz, Lillian D., Ph.D. "What Would You Like to Wear?" *Parents*, February 1990.
Kelly, Paula, M.D., ed. *First-Year Baby Care*. Minn.: Meadowbrook Press, 1989.
Kingsley, Philip. *The Complete Hair Book*. New York: Grosset & Dunlap, 1979.
Levine, Suzanne M., D.P.M. *My Feet Are Killing Me!* New York: Ballantine Books, 1987.
Lewkowicz, David J., Ph.D. "The Five Senses." *Expecting*, Winter 1991–92.
Meier, Barry. "The Slow But Steady Progress in Stopping Tap-Water Burns." *New York Times*, May 5, 1990.
Miller, Jeanne E. *The Perfectly Safe Home*. New York: Fireside, 1991.
Novick, Nelson Lee, M.D. *Baby Skin*. New York: Clarkson N. Potter, 1991.
O'Neill, Catherine. "Watch Out for Scalding Water." *Washington Post*, May 8, 1990.
Phillips, Debora, and Fred Bernstein. *How to Give Your Child a Great Self-Image*. New York: Plume, 1991.
Punches, Laurie. *How to Simply Cut Children's Hair*. South Lake Tahoe, Calif.: Punches Productions, 1989.
Rakow, Phyllis L. " 'Contacting' All Kids!" *Vision Care Assistant*, July/August 1990.
Robins, Perry, M.D. *SunSense*. New York: The Skin Cancer Foundation, 1990.
Schoen, Linda Allen, and Paul Lazar, M.D. *The Look You Like*. New York: Marcel Dekker, Inc., 1990.
Segal, Julius, Ph.D., and Zelda Segal. "Your Child's Body Image." *Parents*, August 1992.
Shanok, Rebecca Shahmoon, Ph.D. "Moving into Puberty." *Parents*, May 1991.
Shelov, Steven P., M.D., and Robert E. Hannemann, M.D., eds. *The American Academy of Pediatrics Caring For Your Baby and Young Child: Birth to Age Five*. New York: Bantam Books, 1991.
Siegel, Mary-Ellen. *Safe in the Sun*. New York: Walker and Company, 1990.
Smolen, Marguerite. "What Does Baby See?" *Expecting*, Winter 1990–91.
———. "The Diaper Decision." *Expecting*, Spring 1992.
Stehlin, Dori. "Cosmetic Allergies." *FDA Consumer*, November 1986.
Sullivan, Barbara. "Beyond the Birthday Suit." *Children's Business*, May 1992.
Tkac, Debora, ed. *The Doctor's Book of Home Remedies*. Emmaus, Pa.: Rodale Press, 1990.
Trevor-Roper, Patrick. *The World Through Blunted Sight*. New York: Bobbs-Merrill Co., 1970.
Yarrow, Leah. "Does Your Child Need Braces?" *Parents*, November 1990.
Zviak, Charles, ed. *The Science of Hair Care*. New York: Marcel Dekker, 1986.

Index

Acetaminophen, 60
Acne, 14–15
Aerosol sprays, 165, 167
Alcohol, 14, 46, 56, 57
Alkaline soaps, 19
Allergies, 13–14, 17, 20, 24, 56, 58
   bath remedies, 47, 48
   bee and wasp sting, 67–68
   and bubble bath, 45
   and poison ivy, 64–66
Aloe vera, 20, 60
Alopecia areata, 87
Alpha-bisabolol, 76
Amblyopia, 144, 146–48, 151, 159
American Academy of Dermatology, 7, 18, 55, 61, 66, 70
American Academy of Ophthalmology, 142, 167
American Academy of Pediatric Dentistry, 113
American Association of Orthodontics, 130, 133
American Dental Association, 119
American Optometric Association, 142, 145, 152, 165
American Podiatric Medical Association, 192–93
Amylase, 126–27
Anagen stage, 73
Anaphylaxis kit, 68
Antibacterial products, 30, 31
Antibiotics, 29, 65, 70
Antifrizz treatment, 84
Antifungal products, 13, 29, 87
Antihistamine, 68
Antiscald devices, 44–45
Antiseptic lotion, 28
Aromatherapy, 47
Astigmatism, 142, 147, 148, 149–50, 162
Athletic shoes, 194
Aveeno, 20

Baby
   bathing, 34, 35–38, 42

Index

Baby (cont'd)
    clothing, 172–74, 176, 181–82, 187, 188
    cuts and scrapes, 30, 31
    dental checkup, 121–22
    eyes, 140–44
    glasses, 156–58
    hair care, 37, 73, 77–78, 90, 91
    insect repellent, 71
    massage, 38–42
    nail care, 26–27
    shoes and boots, 184, 191–92
    skin care, 7–18
    sunburn, 59, 60
    sun protection, 54–55, 56
    teeth and gums, 112–16, 117–18
Baby-bottle tooth decay, 115–16
Baby Magic Lite Baby Oil, 10
Baby Orajel Teething Gel, 114
Baby Orajel Tooth and Gum Cleanser, 113
Baby wash bags, 48
Baby wipes, 11
Baking soda bath, 48
Ballpoint pen ink stain, 195
Bandage, adhesive strip, 31
Bare feet, 68
Barrettes, 110
Basis, 19
Bathing, 27, 34–52
    baby, 7–8, 35–38
    and eczema, 17
    skin check, 61
    soak remedies, 47–49
Bathmat, 43
Bath thermometer, 8
Bausch & Lomb InVision Institute, 162–63
Bee and wasp stings, 67–68
Beech-Nut Baby's First Spring Water, 124
Behavioral therapy, 88
Behavior modification, 29–30
Benzocaine, 60

Benzoyl peroxide solution, 14
Berman, Dr. Marvin, 118
Bibs, 174
Bite plane, 137
Black children, 86
    boy's haircut, 97–98
    girl's haircut, 102–4
    hair styling, 107–8
Bleeding, 30, 31
Blindness, 62
Blisters, 16–18, 59, 64, 65
Blood stains, 195
Blood vessels, 6
Blow-drying hair, 104–5
Body Shop, 9, 48–49
Booties, 174
Boots, 183, 184, 186
Braces, 129–38
Braids, 109. *See also* Cornrows
Brain disorders, 150–51
Breathing, labored, 9
Brushing hair, 90, 91, 110
Bubble bath, 45–46
Bumble & Bumble Salon, 106

Calamine lotion, 65, 69, 70
Calcium, 126
Camphor, 25
Candles, 50
Caswell-Massey shops, 10, 47
Cataracts, 147, 151
Ceramic braces, 134–35
Cerebral palsy, 150
Chamomile, 20, 47, 76
Chemicals, 167
    burns, in eye, 169
Chewing gum
    in hair, 85
    stains, 195
    and teeth, 127
Chicken pox, 20, 48
Chigger bites, 68–69
Children's National Medical Center, 44

Index

Chlorinated water, 75, 84–85
Chocolate stains, 195
Citrus juice stains, 195
Clothing, 171–96
  baby, 172–74
  and color blindness, 152
  organizing, 179, 180–81
  for outdoors, 66, 68, 79
  shopping, 189–91
  stains, 194–96
  stressless dressing, 1, 178–81
Coconut acid, 19
Colds, 22, 23, 25
Cold sore, 25–26
Colic, 38
Collagen, 6
Colloidal oatmeal, 20, 48, 49, 65
Color blindness, 144, 151–53
Colors, newborns and, 141
Comb, 81, 90, 110
Comfrey tea, 47
Complete Healthy Hair Book, The (Kingsley), 77
Compresses, 25–26, 59, 65, 69, 70
Cones, 152
Constipation, 41
Consumer Product Safety Commission (CPSC), 173, 174
Contact lenses, 150, 159–65
Cornea, 140, 148, 160, 162, 163
  scratched, 169
Cornrows, 107–8
Cornstarch, 9, 60
Cortex, hair, 74, 80
Corticosteroids, 65
Cotton, 16, 176, 177, 186–87
  fresh, 33
  sleepwear, 174
Cotton balls, 30, 35–36
Cotton/poly blends, 187
Cowlicks, 109
Cradle cap, 15
Crayon stains, 195

Cuticle, hair, 74, 75–76
Cuticles, nail, 26, 28, 29
Cuts and scrapes, 30–31
  of eye or lid, 169–70
Cyclo-methicone, 10

Dandruff, 15, 86
Davis, Glen, 94
Day, Dr. Susan, 148
Deet (diethyltoluamide), 71
Delirium, 7
Dental care, 111–38
Dental checkups, 121–23, 136–37
Deodorant soaps, 18–19
Dermis, 6
Detangling spray, 80, 91
Detergents, 14, 19
Dextrin, 20
Diabetes, 87
Diaper rash, 11–14, 20, 48
Diapers, 12–13, 14
Diarrhea, 67
Diet, 17, 125, 126–27
Disinfectants, 26
Dove soap, 19–20
Down's syndrome, 150
Dresses, 178
Dry skin, 23–24, 48

Echinacea, 76
Eczema, 16–17, 20, 48
Elastin, 6
Emery board, 27
Emotional trauma, 87–88
Epidermis, 6, 73–74
Epinephrine, 68
Erythromycin, 15, 59
EVA, 189, 194
Eye(s), 139–70. *See also* Glasses; Vision
  baby's, 140–42
  bites near, 69
  checkups, 142–44, 153–54
  infection, 32, 147

Index

Eye(s) (*cont'd*)
  injury, 145, 151, 168–70
  makeup, 32
  patch, 147–48
  problems, 140, 144–53, 159
  safety, 71, 167–68
Eyestrain prevention, 165–67

Fabric softeners, 12, 14
Face, 40
  cleansing, 19, 21–22
  cuts, 31
  makeup and masks, 32–33
Family Focus, Inc., 39
Farsightedness, 144, 147, 148, 149, 151
Faucet safety, 43, 44–45
Fever, 7, 25, 39, 59, 60, 115
Fingerpaint stains, 196
Fireworks, 167
Flexon, 155
Flossing, 113, 120–21, 136
Flu, 22, 70
Fluoride, 123–24
Fluorosis, 117, 124–25
Flynn, Dr. John, 143, 162
Folliculitis, 10
Food and Drug Administration, 45
Fragrances, 14, 19, 68, 69
Frames, 154–56, 157
Freckles, 54, 56

Geranium oil, 47
Ginseng extract, 76
Glasses, 153–59
Gloves, 183
Glycerine soaps, 9, 20
Gordon, Michael, 106
Grape juice stains, 196
Grass stains, 196
Grease stains, 196
Gritty soaps, 19
Grooming, 1, 2
Guns, 167

Hair
  baby, 15, 90
  blow-drying, 104–5
  cleaning, 72–88
  curling and styling, 105–10
  cutting, 89–105
  loss, 87–88
  washing, 77–80
Hair accessories, 91, 109–10
Hair conditioners, 76, 81–82
  for Black hair, 108
Hair follicles, 6, 7, 74, 107
Hair relaxing kits, 108
Hands, 22–23
Hangnails, 28, 29
Hanna Andersson catalog, 185
Hat, 55, 62, 182, 183
  hair, 83
Headbands, 110
Head lice, 85–86
Heat rash, 7, 10
Herpes Simplex Virus (HSV), 25
Hives, 48, 67
Home remedies, 3
  bath soaks, 47–49
  for cold sores, 25–26
  for gum in hair, 85
  for poison ivy, 64–65
  for sunburn, 47, 59–60
  for teething, 114
Hydrocephalus, 150–51
Hydrocortisone cream, 13, 17, 23, 60
Hyperopia. *See* Farsightedness
Hypoallergenic products, 24, 46, 77

Impetigo, 17–18
Injuries
  cuts, 30–31
  eye, 167–72
  teeth, 127–29
Insect
  bites, 48, 68–70
  repellents, 70–71

Index

Interceptive treatment, 131–32
Itching, 20, 48, 65

Jackets, 183–84
Jackson, Judith, 47
Jeans, 175–76, 183
Johnson and Johnson Dental Floss for Kids, 120

Kellner, Jon C., 124
Keratin, 6, 73–74
Kids at Large catalog, 177
Kingsley, Philip, 77, 84

Lands' End catalog, 188
Lanolin, 14, 20
Laundering, 12–13
Lavender oil, 47
Lazy eye. *See* Amblyopia
Leggings, 177
Lens, 140, 146, 147, 148
Lever 2000, 19
Lia Schorr's Seasonal Skin Care (Schorr), 23
Licorice root, 20
Lip balm or ointment, 24–25
Lips, 24–25, 58
Lipstick stains, 196
Liquid Dial, 22
Litman, Ernie, 190
Little Mermaid makeup, 32
Lotions
  baby, 10, 14
  body, 23–24, 28, 49, 68, 84
  sunburn, 60
Lotrimin, 13
Lowila, 20
Lyme disease, 69–70

Makeup, 32
  stains, 196
Malocclusion, 129–30, 131
Manicures, 27
Massage, baby, 38–42

Measles, 48
Medulla, hair, 74
Melanin, 6, 7, 54, 58
Melanoma, 54, 61–62
Milia, 7
Milk, 48, 60, 126
  stains, 195
Mineral oil, 10, 11
Minibraces, 134
Mirror, 141
Mittens, 183
Moisturizers, 19–20, 22
Moles, 61–62
Mosquito bites, 69
Mouth, 71
  guards, 129
Muscle tissue, 6
Mustela Extra Mild Moisturizing Lotion, 10
Myopia. *See* Nearsightedness

Nails, 17, 18, 26–30, 39, 165
  care kit, 27, 28
  ingrown, 27
Nail polish, 29
  stains, 196
National Safe Kids Campaign, 44
Nearsightedness, 144, 146, 147, 148–49, 159, 163
Neutral soaps, 19–20
Neutrogena, 20
Newborn
  acne, 14–15
  clothing, 172–74
  eyesight, 140, 142
  massage, 39
  skin care, 7–8
No-tears baby shampoo, 76
No-tears sunscreen, 57
Nubest & Co. Salon, 94

Oatmeal-based soaps, 17
Oil glands, 6, 7, 74

Index

Oils
  baby, 10, 15, 16, 23, 48
  bath, 47
  for Black hair, 108
  massage, 39–40
Ophthalmologist, 142, 143, 147, 153
Optic nerve disease, 152
Optometrist, 142, 143, 147, 153
Orthodontist, 131–33
OshKosh B'Gosh, 175, 176
Overweight children, 177–78

PABA, 56, 57
Padimate A and O, 56
Paller, Dr. Amy, 23–24
Parent and parenting, 1–4
Paronychia, 29
Patch-testing, 58–59
Paul Mitchell's Baby Don't Cry Shampoo, 76
Pears Soap, 20
Pediatric dentist, 113, 122–24, 130
Pediatric dermatologist, 14, 33, 65
Pediatrician, 13, 14, 16, 26, 27, 29, 30, 31–32, 59, 65, 67, 69, 70, 115, 168, 169
Pediatric ophthalmologist, 143
Perfectly Safe, 44
Periodontic problems, 130
Permanent teeth, 119–20
Perms, 105
Pert Plus for Kids, 76
Petroleum jelly, 10–11, 23, 25, 26
Phenol, 25
Philip Kingsley's Swimcap Cream, 84
Photosensitivity, 59
Pimples, 13, 15
Pincurl set, 107
Plant extracts, 20
Plastic or rubber pants, 12, 14
Poison ivy, oak, and sumac, 20, 64–66
Pomades, 108
Ponchos, 185

Ponytails, 109
Powder, 9, 14, 16
Premature children, 142
Preparation for Birth (Simkin and Savage), 39
Prickly heat, 16, 48
Privacy, 51–52
Pumice, 19
Pus, 28, 29
PVC vinyl, 184, 185, 188, 189

Rainwear, 184–86
Rashes, 7, 10, 11–17, 59, 115
  and bubble bath, 46
  insect and tick bite, 69, 70
  poison ivy, 64–65
Removable appliances, 137–38
Retainer, 137
Retina, 140, 141, 148, 149, 152
Rhus plant family, 64
Rigel, Dr. Darrell S., 58
Rigid lenses, 163
Ringworm, 87
Rods, 152
Ryan, Julie, 162

Safety tips
  bath, 38, 43–44, 46, 48
  eye injury prevention, 167–68
  massage, 39
  shower, 51
  skin, 61
  sleepwear, 174
  sunburn, 60
  water temperature, 44–45
Salt water, 85
Savage, Beverly, 39
Save-a-Tooth, 128
Scalp, 14, 36, 74, 79
  problems, 31, 85–88
Scarring, 32
Scentual Touch (Jackson), 47
Schorr, Lia, 23, 60

Index

Sea Breeze, 28
Sealants, 125–26
Seborrhea, 15
Sebum, 74
Second-degree burn, 59
Self-esteem, 1
   and braces, 131
   and hair, 75, 105, 110
Shampoo, 76–77, 85
   head lice, 86
Shampooing, 32, 77–82
   Black child's hair, 108
   for cradle cap, 15
Shampoo shield, 78
Shock, 7, 67
Shoes, 180, 183, 188–89, 191–94
Shower, 50–51
Simkin, Diana, 39
Skin, 5–33. *See also* Allergies; Sun protection
   baby, 7–18
   bath soaks for, 47–49
   chapped, 23–25
   infection, 15, 17, 28, 29, 31, 65
   and massage, 39
   outdoor care, 54–71
   problems, 11–18, 19, 23–26
   safety check for, 61–62
   tones, and sun, 54, 56
   washing, 18–23
   and water temperature, 44–45
Skin cancer, 54, 61–62
Skin Cancer Foundation, 7, 55, 56, 57, 61
Ski trip, 25
Sleepwear, 174
Smoking, 8
Snacks, 126–27
Snowsuit, 182
Soaps and cleansers, 17, 18–20, 22
   alternative, 19, 48–49
   baby, 8–9
Sodium cocoate, 19

Sodium cocoyl isethionate, 19
Sodium isethionate, 19
Sodium palm kernelate, 19
Sodium tallowate, 19
Soft contact lenses, 161–64
Soft styling rods, 106–7
Split ends, 76
Sponge bath, 35–36
Sprays, 167
Stainless steel braces, 134
Stains, 194–96
Static, 83
Stearic acid, 19
Steroids, 87
Stitches, 31–32
Storrs, Dr. Frances, 12
Strabismus, 140, 142, 144, 146, 147, 150–52
Straightening, hair, 108
Stretchies, 173
Stride-Rite Snow Bank, 184
Stride-Rite Spout, 184
Stride-Rite Two-Step boot, 186
Subcutaneous tissue, 6
Sugar, 116, 126
Summer
   clothing, 186–88
   hair care, 84–85
Sunburn, 20, 47, 48, 59–60
   in infants, 7
Sunglass Association of America, 63
Sunglasses, 62–63
Sunlight, 7, 25, 59, 60, 62, 75, 84
Sun protection, 25, 54–59, 62, 84
   for eyes, 62–63
   newborns and, 7
Sun Protection Factor (SPF), 55, 57, 58
Sunscreen, 25, 55, 56–59, 68, 84
Superfatted soaps, 17, 19
Sweat glands, 5, 6, 7, 10, 19
Sweatshirts and pants, 176–77
Swimsuits, 178, 186, 187–88

Index

Talcum powder, 9
Tangerine oil, 47
Tangles, 76, 80–81, 91
Tayer, Dr. Barton H., 132, 137
Teasing, 156–58
Teeth, 112–29
   baby, 112–16, 119
   braces, 129–38
   injuries, 127–29
Teething, 114–15
Television, 166
Telogen stage, 73
Tetracycline, 59
Thumb Guard, 137
Thumb sucking, 123, 129, 137
Ticks, 69–70
Titanium dioxide, 57
TMJ disorders, 130, 137
Toothbrush, 116–17
Toothpaste, 117, 119, 124
Toric contact lenses, 150, 162–63
Towel, 49
Toxic erythema, 7
Toy safety, 167
Traction alopecia, 109
Triclocarban, 18
Triclosan, 18
T-shirts, 175, 177, 183
Tumors, 147, 151
Turning Heads Salon, 107

Ultraviolet light (UV), 55, 57, 63
Umbilical cord, 36, 39
Unifit bridge, 154–55
Urinary tract infections, 45
Urushiol, 64

Vegetable jelly, 11
Velcro, 176, 180, 184, 193
Vinegar bath, 48
Viruses, 22, 25
Vision, 144–53
   testing, 142–44, 152
Vitamin E-enriched cream, 33

Washing
   clothes, 194–96
   face, 21–22
   hair, 77–80
   hands, 22–23
   soap for, 8–9, 18–20
Waterproof v. water-resistant fabrics, 183, 184, 185
   sunscreens, 57
Water temperature, 44–45
Weather, 179
Weber, Dr. Jack, 62
Wheezing, 9, 67
Whiteheads, 7, 13, 14, 15
Winter
   clothes, 181–84
   hair care, 82–83
Wippette Kids, 185
Witch hazel, 26

X rays, dental, 122–23

Yeast infection, 13
Yogurt, 33, 60

Zinc oxide cream, 13, 57
Zippers, 173, 184, 190